*Simon & Schuster*

*New York  London  Toronto*

*Sydney  Tokyo  Singapore*

# Benson Bobrick

# Knotted Tongues

*Stuttering in History*

*and the Quest*

*for a Cure*

SIMON & SCHUSTER
Rockefeller Center
1230 Avenue of the Americas
New York, New York 10020
Copyright © 1995 by Benson Bobrick
Illustrations copyright © 1994 by Marco Hernandez
All rights reserved, including the right of reproduc-
tion in whole or in part in any form.
SIMON & SCHUSTER and colophon are registered
trademarks of Simon & Schuster Inc.
Designed by Karolina Harris
Manufactured in the United States of America
1 3 5 7 9 10 8 6 4 2
Library of Congress Cataloging-in-Publication Data
Bobrick, Benson, date.
Knotted tongues: stuttering in history and the quest
for a cure/Benson Bobrick.
p.    cm.
Includes bibliographical references and index.
1. Stuttering. 2. Stuttering—History. 3. Stuttering—
Case studies. I. Title.
RC424.B637    1995
616.85'54—dc20                    94-32429
                                    CIP


ISBN: 978-1-5011-4087-7


"Stutterer," © 1961, 1962, 1968, 1972, 1973, 1974,
1983 by Alan Dugan. From *New and Collected Poems*
by Alan Dugan, first published by The Ecco Press in
1983. Reprinted by permission.

*To Jim*

*(il miglior interlocutore)*

# Prefatory Note and Acknowledgments

What used to be known academically as dysphemia is called stammering in Great Britain and stuttering in the United States. In current clinical usage, the two are identical terms. And they are so used in this book.

Like all books, mine has an ideal reader: one interested in the history of a medical conundrum and its impact on people's lives. Some of the people are famous, but my larger purpose (at which I hope all sympathetic readers will connive) is not biographical but to help educate the public about one of the most perplexing disorders affecting mankind.

The help I have received cannot be adequately expressed by a mere reiteration of thanks; but I would be unpardonably remiss if I did not gratefully name: Catherine Otto, who generously gave of her time, encouragement, and advice, as well as access to her files; Alison Garvin-Cullen, my undaunted therapist some years back under Catherine Otto's direction; Eric Warren, friend and articulate exemplar; John Ahlbach, director of the National Stuttering Project (whose monthly newsletter is a mine of pertinent information); Ronald L. Webster of the Hollins Communications Research Institute in Roanoke, Virginia, whose research and therapeutic approach have been on the cutting edge; Diana Rodriguez, from whom I acquired a better understanding over time of certain aspects of the disorder; Edward Hoagland and Harold Brodkey, who graciously allowed me to interview them at some length; Valerie Traina, who was diligent and resourceful in helping with early research; and Hilary Bloom, who took a loving (if sometimes maddeningly critical) interest in the manuscript as it evolved. I am also indebted to the staffs of the New York Public Library, the Library of the New York Academy of Medicine, the Butler, Biology, and Health Sciences Libraries of Columbia University, and to numerous organizations that steered material my way, including the American Speech-Language Hearing Association, the Institute for Stuttering Treatment and Research in Alberta, Canada, the International Fluency Association, the National Council on Stuttering, the National Institute of Neurological and Communicative Disorders, Speak Easy of Canada, the Speak Easy International Foundation, the Stuttering Foundation of America, and the Stuttering Research Foundation. My agent, Russell Galen, and Elaine Pfefferblit of Simon & Schuster, did much to nourish the book by their belief in it at the outset; I am especially grateful to my editor, Bob Bender, for his care, commitment, and enlightened indulgence in allowing me to revise the manuscript to my heart's content. The efforts of Johanna Li, his capable assistant, and Isolde C. Sauer, the copy editing supervisor, also merit thanks.

"Lord, open my breast," said Moses,
"and do Thou ease for me my task,
Unloose the knot upon my tongue,
that they may understand my words."
—*Koran,* 20:26–29

# Contents

# Part One

## Anatomy
## of Melancholy

# Chapter One

Of words, and the murder of words, he dreamed,
Whose very syllables are the sounds of fears.

These are the only lines I can remember now from a poem I wrote when I was about nineteen about Caedmon, the tongue-tied Anglo-Saxon poet, whose speech was freed by an angel who appeared to him in a dream. Notwithstanding my passion at the time for early English verse, the poem's dark wellspring was my own experience with stuttering; and although I suppose I was past believing in a divine or miraculous cure, I do remember that my poem ended with a prayer.

The experience of stuttering has sometimes been compared to wandering without bearings through a maze or desert wilderness or trackless wood: "You know there is a way out, but you can't seem to find it. You try, but you only go in circles and end up more lost than you were before."

It wasn't until I was thirty-eight years old that I found a path into the clear.

This book is an account of one of the great conundrums of medical history—"the most complex disorganization of functioning," in the words of one authority, "in the field of medicine and psychiatry." It also explores the impact of stuttering on the lives of various notable men and women, its social profile, the current clinical outlook, and the author's own successful quest for deliverance.

Many more men than women stutter, and so I hope it will be allowed if, for convenience, I generally refer to the stutterer as "he." "The girl imprisoned in the tower of a stammer" (as W. H. Auden and Christopher Isherwood put it in their early verse drama, *The Ascent of F6*) is no less miserable, of course, and the quaint adage of the Roman poet Horace—"Feminas verba balba decent"—that stuttering is becoming in a woman, referred more to shyness in utterance than to the malady itself. Almost no one stutters deliberately, although down through the ages the affectation of a slight stutter or lisp has been cultivated occasionally as a sign of gentility. Ovid in the *Art of Love* noted that such affectations were current in his day among Roman girls. But in commenting upon such notions, James Hunt, one of the best of the nineteenth-century therapists, remarked, "Some may imagine that a slight singularity of enunciation draws attention to other graces a young lady may possess, but certain it is that confirmed stuttering throws all the enchantments of youth and beauty into the shade, and must eventually blight her happiness."

Moses, Demosthenes, Vergil, Charles I, Charles Lamb,

Lewis Carroll, W. Somerset Maugham, Henry James, Winston Churchill, and Marilyn Monroe were all afflicted, merely among the notables, along with countless others down through the ages of far more modest repute. Two and a half million Americans—fifty-five million people worldwide—stutter; and though their baffling malady has been subjected to confident analysis for over twenty-five hundred years, most endure it without hope of cure. In the United States and elsewhere, no unified program of experimental therapy yet exists, presenting a bizarre diversity of options—most of them ineffectual—to those in need.

Symptomatically defined in brief as involuntary repetitions or prolongations of sounds with blocking or other spasmodic interruptions in the rhythmical flow of speech, stuttering may, from case to case, include blinking and other facial tics, tremors of the lips and jaw, gasping, stamping of the feet, jerking of the head, contortions of the whole body, and even foaming at the mouth as in an epileptic fit.

Though no one stutters all the time, and every stutterer is capable of fluent asides, in the vivid daily anticipation of glottal catastrophe, the disorder is apt to dominate the victim's social and emotional life.

Roughly one hundred muscles are smoothly coordinated in the normal (and normally automatic), simple act of speech. The poet Alan Dugan has masterfully evoked the complex ordeal that can result when their timing goes awry:

> Courage: your tongue has left
> its natural position in the cheek
> where eddies of the breath
> are navigable calms. Now
> it locks against the glottis or

is snapped at by the teeth,
in mid-stream: it must be work
to get out what you mean:
the rapids of the breath
are furious with belief
and want the tongue, as blood
and animal of speech,
to stop it, block it or come clean
over the rocks of teeth
and down the races of the air,
tumbled and bruised to death.
Relax it into acting, be
the air's straw-hat
canoeist with a mandolin
yodeling over the falls.
This is the sound advice
of experts and a true despair:
it is the toll to pass the locks
down to the old mill stream
where lies of love are fair.

The "sound advice of experts" notwithstanding, the therapeutic history of stuttering has been astonishing. Demosthenes was obliged to labor up steep inclines with lead plates strapped to his chest and to declaim over the roar of the ocean with pebbles in his mouth. Ancient physicians prescribed everything from blistering afflicted tongues to wrapping them in little towels. In the Middle Ages, bloodletting and powerful cathartics were often applied, and searing irons to the lips. One American Indian tribe obliged stutterers to recite "I give my stuttering to you" to a board with a knothole in it, then to spit through the hole to get the devil out of their throats. Johann Amman, a seventeenth-century Swiss physician, recommended gymnastic exercises for the lips and jaw, and a French specialist by the name of Jean Marc Itard invented a little fork made out of gold or ivory to support the tongue during speech. The Prussian botanist and surgeon J. F. Dieffenbach diagnosed a lingual cramp and cut a triangular wedge from the base of the tongue. The common houseplant dieffenbachia, known colloquially as dumbcane, indicates the practical effect of his surgery.

At one time or another, stuttering has also been popularly traced to childhood trauma, sibling rivalry, suppressed anger, infantile sexual fixations, deformations of the tongue, lips, palate, jaw, or larynx, chemical (or humoral) imbalance, strict upbringing, vicious habit, guilt, approach–avoidance conflicts, and so on, and treated by biofeedback, hypnosis, operant conditioning, electric shock, faith healing, drugs, and of course psychoanalysis. Mounting clinical evidence today, however, indicates that stuttering is, after all, an inheritable, physically based problem involving a neurological defect in the auditory feedback loop, perhaps specifically pertaining to anomalies of sound transmission through the skull.

# Chapter Two

Robert Burton in his compendious *Anatomy of Melancholy,* published in 1621, singled out stuttering as one of melancholy's "soonest" causes—which may be counted some kind of privilege in a work that in learned and hilarious fashion finds melancholy in just about everything under the sun. At the time, melancholy was actually a kind of biochemical term (connected with the doctrine of the four humors), but its manifestations in Burton's symptomatic definition were "anguish of mind" accompanied by "sorrow and fear." In any case, a diagnostic link between the two belonged to a long and august tradition that could be traced back to Aristotle and that threads its way without dissent through the early Christian and medieval eras, past Burton down to modern times. In 1842, the great speech pathologist

Karl Ludwig Merkel, who stuttered himself, observed that stutterers naturally tend toward "a certain reserve, absorption, inclination to solitude and to contemplation, that can even develop into melancholy, if nourished by temperament." And Charles Dickens, who wrote an article on stammering in 1856 for the popular weekly *Household Words,* remarked: "Stammering [in a child] rises as a barrier by which the sufferer feels that the world without is separated from the world within."

How could it be otherwise? Stuttering is an affliction that renders defective the uniquely human capacity for speech. In its severest form, it can be a crippling disability; and of all disabilities, it is perhaps the least understood. The dignity of the person, his distinctive humanity, and even his soul, as made manifest in rational discourse, was (and is) by tradition associated with speech. Together with the capacity for thought that it expresses through language, speech defines us as human more adequately than any other faculty we have. Its deprivation—in stuttering, its audible and visible disintegration—cannot but be felt as a catastrophe.

In the Biblical account of Man's creation in Genesis (2:19), speech is Adam's first and quintessential human act. "And out of the ground the Lord God formed every beast of the field, and every fowl of the air; and brought them unto Adam to see what he would call them: and whatsoever Adam called every living creature, that was the name thereof." Early Greek philosophy regarded speech as "the conversation of the soul." Speech is "the stream of thought moving outward from the soul to the lips," we may read in the *Sophist,* one of the Platonic dialogues; and Aristotle (who raised—and answered—many of the same questions we continue to mull over about apes and dolphins) similarly understood speech as an expression of the soul or mind. Upon Aristotle's belief, the Stoic philosophers were to build their concept of speech as a manifestation of the logos, the divinely ordering principle implicit in the cosmos or Creation. In Cicero's dialogue *On the Nature of the Gods,* the faculty of speech is also said to be the foundation of civilized society. These threads came together in the Gospel According to St. John where the Word, "in the beginning," was associated both with the logos and (in ways incomparably more powerful) with its incarnation in a Redeemer at the end of Time. The eradication of stuttering, it may be noted, is one of the afflictions specifically associated in Isaiah 32 with the redemption of the world.

In short, the soul on earth reflected the light of the divine idea, and speech the light of the soul. It was therefore "not just a physical function." While other bodily ills were attended to by "earthly" physicians, the priest was uniquely qualified, on occasion, to intervene as speech therapist. And so he does in the Venerable Bede's account of a miraculous cure effected by the seventh-century Bishop John of Hexham:

> In a village not far distant lived a dumb youth known to the bishop; for he had often visited him to receive alms and had never been able to utter a single word. In addition, he had so many scabs and scales on his head that no hair ever grew on the crown, but only a few wisps stood up in a ragged circle round it. So the bishop ordered this youth to be fetched, and a little hut to be made for him in the enclosure round the house where he could live and receive his daily allowance. When one week of Lent was past, on the following Sunday

John told the poor lad to come to him, and when he had entered he ordered him to put out his tongue and show it to him; then he took him by the chin, and making the sign of the holy cross on his tongue, told him to retract it and speak. "Pronounce some word," he said: "say *yea.*" The lad's tongue was loosed, and at once he did what he was told. The bishop then proceeded to the names of letters: "Say A." And he said "A." "Now say B," he said, which the youth did. And when he had repeated the names of each of the letters after the bishop, the latter added syllables and words for him to repeat after him. When he had uttered every word accordingly, the bishop set him to repeat longer sentences, and he did so. All those who were present say that all that day and the next night, as long as he could keep awake, the youth never stopped saying something and expressing his own inner thoughts and wishes to others, which he had never been able to do previously.

As for his other maladies (such as the scabs on his crown), they were referred to the village doctor.

The Renaissance accepted the divinity of speech as a reflection of the soul even while exploring its anatomical operation; and since the physical habitation of the soul was thought to be the mind, theories about the cerebral control of speech functions did not of themselves contradict the sacred idea. Today, of course, speech is no longer theologized in the same way, since it has become the domain of linguistics; but powerful evidence (via Chomsky and others) that grammar may be inborn lends support to the notion that the human capacity for language is not shared, even remotely, by any other living form.

So far as we know, even the most intelligent animals communicate at best by signs (gesture or voice), with direct reference to some immediate object or circumstance. Human beings, on the other hand, form sounds into words that, in their capacity as symbols, can represent things in their absence, as well as abstract thoughts. The capacity for abstraction makes articulate speech possible, and the evolution of speech and thought are evidently joined. This is illustrated by the fact that little children talk to themselves and think aloud. The talent for mimicry shown by certain birds, the vocalization and gestures of other mammals, the signs and sounds of dolphins and apes, are simply not speech in the same sense. *Homo loquens,* or "Speaking Man," as one historian remarks, may after all be our "most satisfactory appellation." One Byzantine monk, Meletius, of the Monastery of the Holy Trinity in Asia Minor, supposed the Greek word for man *(anthropos)* derived from a phrase meaning "one who utters articulate voice." Although not the best etymologist, he may not, in principle, have been entirely wrong. Speech, it seems, is bound up with our very humanity.

This finds confirmation in anatomy. From the moment we are born our vocal apparatus undergoes an evolution that uniquely suits it for articulate speech. In the beginning, the child's larynx is positioned high in the throat (like that of most apes and other mammals), allowing it to breathe and swallow at the same time. It can do so because the larynx divides the throat into two separate channels, to facilitate suckling. For a similar reason, the epiglottis is more superiorly placed, with its tip close to the soft palate, and the tongue forward in the mouth. Over time, however (usually in the second year of life), the larynx begins to descend until the two channels cross. Eating becomes a bit more perilous, but

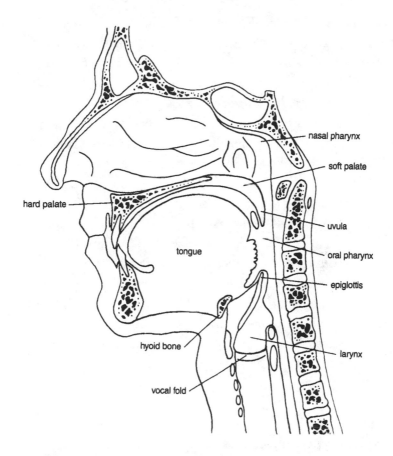

a resonating chamber or pharyngeal area of space is created in the throat that can take sounds that are produced within the larynx and modify them to an extent no other creature can match. To accommodate this chamber, the base of the human skull is uniquely bent.

Meanwhile, in the respiratory system, the diaphragmatic breathing of the infant undergoes changes to include use of the chest, and from the age of two the rib cage expands to accommodate expanding lungs. By age seven, mature breathing patterns have been established; the tongue, half again as large, has been retracted; the size of the larynx has grown considerably; and the upper vocal tract has assumed the double-barreled configuration of maturity.

Language development accompanies anatomy. Speech begins with the birth cry; differentiated crying develops after the first month; and by the third the infant is normally babbling. Vowels are followed by consonants in a sequence possibly related to the change from nursing to the eating of semisolid food. By the end of the first year, the child is usually imitating sounds he hears others make, and (whether he understands them or not) has begun to pronounce single words. Soon thereafter disconnected words are combined into rudimentary sentences (in what we call "baby talk"), and from then on his linguistic development steadily matures. By the age of five to seven, with all three speech systems—for respiration, voicing, and articulation—in place, he can begin to talk (in the physiological sense) like an adult.

Speech sounds are "vibrations that occur in air." The air is provided by a bellows-like respiratory apparatus; and the sounds are shaped in the breath stream by the movement and vibrations of the vocal cords and the positions the articulators assume in modifying the vocal tract. The vocal cords are two small muscular folds located in the larynx that are brought together during phonation, and part for respiration; the space between, or glottis (Greek for "tongue"), is the origin of voice. The vocal tract, above the larynx, consists of the oral and nasal cavities and the articulators (tongue, lips, jaw) within the mouth. In short, the larynx acts as a sound generator; the pharynx as a resonator; and the articulators in the oral cavity as a sound modifier, by which the sounds are transformed into intelligible speech.

Speech is the most finely balanced and complex neuro-muscular activity we possess. It involves coordination of numerous major organs as well as an intricate network of tiny peripheral muscles that instantly intermesh. The number and complexity of the processes to be timed properly in the control of fluent speech is daunting. In one expert description:

> the sentential system for controlling the sequencing of words in sentences; the phonologic system for controlling the sequencing of syllables and phonemes within words; and the muscle movement system for controlling and coordinating the laryngeal, respiratory, and articulatory muscles for producing speech sounds. Moreover, the processes within each of these systems are extremely complex. Considering only the lowest level of speech musculature, over 100 different muscles may be involved in producing a single word, and each must get its appropriate nervous impulses at the required moment in the sequence if the word is to be spoken without disruption.

The average person speaks between one hundred twenty and one hundred eighty words a minute, producing six hundred different vocal tract shapes in that brief time. "That's a lot of behavior," one speech pathologist remarks, "and a lot can go wrong."

A recent report by the U.S. Public Health Service described stuttering as an enigma. It then added (somewhat enigmatically) that everyone seems to know what it sounds like, even if they can't agree as to its cause. Actually, it sounds like a number of things it is not, which is not something everybody knows. To begin with, it has little to do with the vocal fumbling that sometimes occurs when someone is flustered, apoplectically angry, or caught off guard. It is also not the same as neurogenic or "acquired stuttering" (e.g. aphasia), which is associated with head injury or stroke. Nor is it to be confused with "cluttering," which is characterized by rapid, sloppy, jumbled speech in which (with some repetitions and omissions) half-articulated words "pile up like typewriter keys."

Genuine or developmental stuttering emerges in childhood (usually between the ages of two and seven) when a child begins to develop muscle coordination and practice language skills. Because of the normal disfluencies in a young child's speech—hesitations, syllable repetitions, vocalizations between words, and the like—it is sometimes difficult to tell whether the disorder is present or not. Such hesitations usually occur on whole syllables or words, rather than initial sounds, and are as normal as an infant's first awkward steps. However, any frequent repetitions accompanied by signs of tension or struggle, or any apprehension about speaking, is a sign that the disorder has begun to take hold. If at this stage the child is made self-conscious about his speech through anxious or imperious correction, his attempts to acquire the skill may hopelessly fail.

Stuttering involves a loss of control of the speech apparatus. Its primary characteristics (blockings, prolongations or repetitions of sound) are often less conspicuous than its secondary manifestations, which range from subtle gestures to whole body convulsions in an effort to release or complete a sound. Interjections like "well," "er," "ah," "um," and so on may also recur like verbal tics. Henry James used such interjections constantly; Lewis Carroll's upper lip often trembled; the writer Edward Hoagland (by his own description) used to "snort like a rhinoceros" and spit; and the writer John Updike, who devotes an interesting chapter to his own stutter in *Self-Consciousness: Memoirs,* vividly describes the onset of an episode of his own as viewed on tape: "I see the repulsive symptoms of an approaching stammer take possession of my face—an electronically rapid flutter of the eyelashes, a distortion of the mouth as of a leather purse being cinched, a terrified hardening of the upper lip, a fatal tensing and lifting of the voice." Such struggle behaviors may not always be clearly present; however, "a paroxysm of stuttering," as the distinguished Harvard surgeon, Edward Warren, remarked in an article published in the *American Journal of Medical Science* in 1837,

> is formidable to behold. The countenance of the patient is horribly distorted, inarticulate and dissonant sounds issue from his mouth; he will tear his hair, stamp as if with rage, and practise all the gestures of a madman. Even in less violent cases, the whole nervous system is in violent agitation, every nerve in his body, to the ends of his fingers and his toes, seems to him to vibrate, like the strings of a harp, producing a sensation like that caused by the filing of a saw, and he feels a sense of suffocation at his chest. . . .

Many stutterers, in fact, have chronic pains in their chest due to prolonged efforts to speak on residual air. Updike has suggested that most spasms occur "when in truth we are out of breath, when in our haste and anxiety we have forgotten to breathe. Taking a breath, or concentrating on keeping the breath flowing, erases the problem as easily as mist wiped from a windowpane." However, he adds, wisely: "breathing is not necessarily easy. It is one of those physical acts on the edge of thought. . . ." J. S. Greene and E. J. Wells, two physicians associated early in this century with the National Hospital for Speech Disorders, described correct breathing rather nicely in their useful book, *The Cause and Cure of Speech Disorders,* published in 1927:

> The human body is divided into two chambers, an upper and a lower. . . . Air flows in and out of the upper chamber, which contains the lungs, but the compression and expansion take place in the lower chamber and are caused by the rising and falling of the diaphragm. This lower chamber is like a rubber ball, alternately squeezed and released. Many people in taking a deep breath protrude the chest and elevate the shoulders, which causes a tension of the muscles of the neck and throat where the vocal cords are located and a tightness around the nose and mouth. The vocal machine cannot operate properly when subjected to this tension. When breathing correctly for speech there should be no motion at all above the abdomen and only an easy expansion and contraction there. The mouth is open all the time.
>
> The reason that many people find the simple act of speech so exhausting is because they try to force the words out instead of allowing them to come out naturally. The muscles of the throat, neck and face being tense and rigid, the breathing becomes labored and the voice harsh and rasping, all the life and warmth being squeezed out of the words by the muscles of the throat as they issue forth.

During a severe block, both sets of laryngeal muscles contract as hard as they can, virtually paralyzing the vocal cords;
stutterers have been known almost to black out on such occasions, and may cease almost to breathe. One afflicted
physician recalled: "My first morning on the ward I walked
to the nurses' station to introduce myself to the head nurse. I
stuttered badly. My face turned red, the veins in my neck
bulged, my eyes closed, and my head bent over in secondary
struggle behavior as I tried to break the block. Unfortunately, the head nurse did not realize what was happening
and overreacted. Before I knew it, she had pushed me to the
floor, and, as two other nurses pinned my arms and legs
down, she tried to force a plastic airway down my throat."
On another occasion, when consulting a fellow doctor at the
bedside of a patient, he found himself unable to speak, and
the patient had "to explain his own disease."

Some kind of physical jarring may help shake the sound
loose. Children, not knowing quite what speech is, sometimes think the word itself is literally stuck in their mouths.
They may "jump up and down to try to force it out," as in
the case of one little girl who tried try to "squeeze the words
out of her mouth by pressing her hand against her cheek."
And there is the story a therapist tells of a child "who could
release herself from a block only by pulling a hair out of her
head. Though she was only seven," he wrote, "she appeared
to be going bald." Like any result that depends entirely upon
sensation, however, a progressively stronger stimulus is required. There was a student at Harvard, for example, who
discovered one day that he could break his blocks by stamping on the floor. It worked for a while, we are told, but then
he found he had to stamp harder and longer to release a

word. Finally, "the whole house in which he lived seemed to shake from his pounding."

Although stuttering is seldom amusing (at least to stutterers), most can appreciate, in retrospect, how peculiar on occasion their behavior must have seemed. By way of illustration, Patrick Campbell, a British television personality and humorist, recounted the following episode from his own life:

[My stammer] has assumed in its time a wide variety of different forms, and the ability to change its nature without warning. For instance, I used to have for several weeks at a time what I came to call the "muted gibbon" cry. It used to go, "May I awah awah awah awash my ahah ahah ahah ahah ahands please?"

At a formal dinner party, a particularly dynamic form of this stammer made its debut. At this time I was having the muted gibbon call, with rotation. That is, my head turned ponderously from right to left, and then back again, with the effort of speech. It humped the muscles of my neck like a bison, and, in fact, rendered any attempt at articulation completely out of the question.

But I threw myself into it. I set myself to say, "I went bathing yesterday and the water was as warm as toast." I became locked at once. My head turned slowly to the left, the rich blood already pounding into my face. I met the terrified gaze of the diplomat's wife, tried to smile at her, emitted three "ahah ahah ahah's" instead, and then found myself centered upon Theodore (another stammerer, but one who prefaced his attempted speech with a whistle), immediately opposite me. To my absolute consternation I saw that he was busy too. The fool had thrown himself into speech as well, and was now whistling away in short, piercing trills, with his eyes clamped firmly shut. My head ground round to the right. "I awah awah awent . . ." I said to the brisk matron, and then my head started its journey back again. I caught a glimpse of Mrs. Gilbert out of the corner of my eye. Her lips were moving in prayer. I had time to think that she was lucky to have them moving at all, when I became based upon Theodore once more. He must have played the whole of *The Bluebells of Scotland* by this time, but was as far away as ever from saying anything.

It went on through all eternity—some of the guests leaning forward with bright smiles and the perspiration running down their faces, others suddenly exhibiting nervous mannerisms of their own, twitching or plucking at their clothes, or coughing loudly, but all waiting to hear what either Theodore or I might have to add to the fund of human knowledge. Mrs. Gilbert broke it down in the end. Her voice, when she found it, came out in a scream, but . . . she'd done it. In another moment, the whole lot of them were chattering away again.

For all the contortions the afflicted go through, there is, in fact, within the range of normal speech, no such thing per se as a "difficult sound." Nevertheless, past difficulties become associated with memories of failure, and over time every stutterer tends to acquire a list of sounds or words that he becomes convinced are hard to say. As with Campbell, these sounds may constantly change. Moreover, stutterers are differently affected by different speech situations. Some have more difficulty with strangers, others with familiar friends; some more in conversation, others with reading aloud. But almost all dread the telephone, where they are reduced to a voice and their speech is most exposed. The hardest word that most stutterers ever have to pronounce is their name—

not, perhaps, because it has to do with their identity (as is often said) but because it is *inescapably* the word they most often have to say. And to hesitate to say it, to appear even for a moment not to know it, risks making the speaker appear an imbecile. On no word is there more pressure for instant articulation; on no other vocal failure hangs such a social penalty and cost.

One soldier who admitted to being a stutterer (he "came out" in an army publication) described the sudden approach of a feared word this way: "Think of yourself on the highway. It's dark. You're in a hurry. No traffic. You squeeze on the gas. Suddenly, out of nowhere, directly in front of you, looms the terrifying back of a huge truck. You slam on the brakes, spin the wheel, swerve, pray. Anything to keep from colliding. . . . You can't always tell what word it will be. . . . And this breeds the latent terror, the fear that you may blow in a critical moment. Like freezing on words like 'duck' or 'watch out.'"

(Unfortunately, his confession probably didn't put his fellow soldiers much at ease.)

Kindred apprehensions are more subtly acknowledged in the work of the English poet Philip Larkin, who began to stutter at the age of four. In his own description, he tended to have trouble on words beginning with vowels rather than consonants (which is unusual), and "there was no obvious reason for it: no left-handedness or physical accidents. If I had some deep traumatic experience I've forgotten it." From about the age of thirty-five on, he spoke more easily, but relapses were frequent, especially with fatigue or when "confronted by a stammering situation," like having to deal with a postal clerk. Larkin's terror of situations in which speaking could not be avoided found its way *sub rosa* into one of his most somber poems, "Next, Please." Although obviously about disappointed hopes and the inevitability of death and extinction, the poem's title phrase was one he had dreaded hearing as a child, for it signaled his imminent obligation to speak once he reached the head of a line.

To avoid a verbal crack-up, stutterers often scan ahead obsessively for sounds and syllables they dread. If one is encountered but no synonym comes readily to mind, they may reconstruct the entire sentence to express an analogous, comparable, or even very different thought. As a result, their sentences may become, in one description, "elaborate, stilted, pedantic, or Germanic" with the word choices forming "a pattern of dependent probability" like the random variables in a statistical chain. In his sometimes tortuous attempts at conversation, this happened on occasion to Henry James.

A less extreme but still artful example is presented by the physician and theatrical director Jonathan Miller, who once described himself as a skilled paraphraser—a talent he was obliged to develop rather early in life. In an interview, he recalled that when he was growing up in London his parents used to have to give him extra bus fare because he couldn't pronounce his stop. His stop was Marble Arch, which unfortunately began with the same letter as his last name—a problem sound. One day, as the conductor approached, Miller quickly said, "Here's the fare for the arch that is made of marble." When he undertook to narrate *The Body in Question,* his literate and entertaining history of medicine for a three-part television series, he omitted reference to several important figures because he couldn't pronounce their names.

In *A Walker in the City,* the writer Alfred Kazin relates, "I could never say anything except in the most roundabout way; I was a stammerer. . . . I could never seem to get the easiest words out with the right dispatch, and [at school] would often miserably signal from my desk that I did not know the answer rather than get up to stumble and fall and crash on every word. . . . The word that for others was so effortless and so neutral, so unburdened, so simple, so exact, I had first to meditate in advance, to see if I could make it, like a plumber fitting together odd lengths and shapes of pipe."

Not every stutterer yields to this impulse. Edward Hoagland, for example, despite the tenacity of his blocks, rather determinedly resisted word substitution on the grounds that it tended to "bleach out" the personality of his language, "making it bland."

Whether the disorder is conspicuous or not is seldom a true measure of its severity, since (like an iceberg) the submerged portion of fear that attends it is often much greater than its manifestations in other respects. Although many adepts "are able," in Charles Van Riper's words, "to pose as normal speakers," yet "the nervous strain and vigilance necessary to avoid and disguise their symptoms often create stresses so severe as to produce profound emotional breakdowns."

The fact that a stutterer cannot always tell when or why he will have difficulty makes it all the harder to bear. It is this inconsistency, this baffling variability, that is most demoralizing, and keeps him helplessly oscillating between hope and despair. Since, objectively, he can find no excuse for his failure except a seeming hesitation in his speech, he cannot understand why his most gallant efforts fail. Beyond the inevitable toll on self-confidence this takes, its profounder peril is to sow doubt that the will has power at all. James Hunt, the nineteenth-century therapist, reported that some of his patients came to suppose themselves under a mysterious curse, or demonically possessed. Herman Melville (in a more metaphysical way) invoked this suggestion of malevolent involvement in *Billy Budd,* where he describes Billy's "liability" to stutter—his hero's one imperfection—as "a striking instance that the arch interferer, the envious marplot of Eden" always manages "to slip in his little card."

A more impersonal malevolence (in which the devil is supplanted by a kind of neoclassical concept of fate) was imagined by the English novelist Margaret Drabble, who stuttered so badly as a child that she could "hardly speak." As a result, she was virtually friendless, and the frustration she experienced perhaps predisposed her to a fatalistic view of life. In any case, her characters inhabit a balefully malicious universe in which free will exists, if it exists at all, as a more or less inconsequential force in opposition to the divine engines of unhappiness and grief. Undeserved evils and misfortunes beset them, and ultimately oblige their submission to Necessity. In her own life, repeated and apparently inexplicable breakdowns in her speech evidently reinforced her feeling over time that "the axe was always about to fall."

The variability of stuttering also accounts for the popular notion that it may be some sort of deliberate stratagem— used to evoke sympathy, attract attention, dominate a conversation, and so on. The actor James Earl Jones recalls that because he seemed as a boy to talk at times well enough, his family and friends "often accused me of lying about my inability to speak." It wasn't until he entered high school and came under the compassionate tutelage of Stanley E. Crouch, a former college professor who had come out of retirement to teach at the local school, that he discovered he could read aloud effectively from a script. The writer Harold Brodkey, who stutters mildly himself, told this author that he used his own hesitations for thoughtful pauses when he could, but consciously manipulated stuttering is, in the larger sense, relatively rare.

Indeed, although Honoré de Balzac's fictional Père Grandet sometimes faked a stutter to gain advantage in business negotiations, in "real life" there is the decidedly exceptional case of Harold Adrian (Kim) Philby, the British double agent and Soviet master spy.

Philby, the Third Man in the Cambridge spy ring that included Guy Burgess and Donald Maclean was, however duplicitous, evidently a man of intelligence and charm. His wife, Eleanor, an American journalist who married him in Beirut, presented this affectionate (if disingenuous) portrait of him in her autobiography:

> [Kim was] a most attentive husband and an extremely easy man to live with. In spite of his occasional stutter, which some people mistook for repressed violence, he was not at all tense or restless. . . . He was a domesticated, civilized man who enjoyed reading and listening to music. Sometimes he read German poetry to me in his melodious voice, when his stutter disappeared and he sounded like a different person. Cooking was his great hobby and he liked nothing better than to spend three hours in the kitchen preparing an elaborate curry or a boeuf en daube.

In the course of his government career, he held a number of sensitive posts, but during his tenure as first secretary of the British embassy in Washington, D.C., he came under suspicion and was recalled to London to answer charges after the defections to Moscow of Burgess and Maclean. One of his biographers describes the interrogation that took place:

> The trial was held at MI5 headquarters in Leconfield House, Curzon Street, Mayfair, in November 1952. . . . The officer detailed to conduct what MI5 chose to call "a judicial inquiry" was Helenus Milmo, later a King's Counsel and a judge, who had worked for MI5 during the war as an interrogator. His bluff, forceful manner had won him the nickname "Buster." His approach to Philby was to attempt to bully him into a confession.
>
> From the beginning it was apparent that this was not going to work. Milmo needed rapid-fire questions and rapid-fire answers to corner his quarry. Philby fell back on his intermittent stammer to slow the cross-examination to a pace to suit him. In 1968 *The Sunday Times* spoke with an MI5 officer who was present at the inquiry and he gave this hypothetical example of the type of exchange that drove Milmo to fury. Milmo: "Was it a fine day?" Philby: "Yes." Milmo (pouncing). "How do you know?" Philby: "Well . . . there wwwas a temperature of about ffffifty-eight degrees, I suppose. And there wwwas a ssssslight wind from the sssouth. It sssseems to me that constitutes a fffffine day."

Philby was released, and Harold Macmillan, England's prime minister, even issued a public apology in an effort to clear his name. A decade later, however, the net closed around him again, and in 1963 he escaped to Moscow, where he recently died.

In his youth, Philby had been inhibited by his stutter from participating in student debates, and as an adult often relied in getting through a conversation on an elaborate kind of fumbling with his matches and pipe. Any kind of distraction (including "acting") may in fact help, since self-consciousness is a component of the malady; and so stutterers find all sorts of ways of distracting themselves. They may cough, swallow, or clear their throat, spell a word before pronouncing it, interject sudden, swift asides to try to lubricate the flow of words, or rush their speech in some unnatural way in an effort to carry their voice through a feared sound. "Any mechanism," observes Updike, "which displaces your customary voice . . . - eliminates the stoppage; the captive tongue is released into *Maskenfreiheit,* the freedom conferred by masks." Examples abound. Marilyn Monroe's breathy and alluring voice was originally "an attempt to avoid stuttering rather than to sound sexy. She stuttered badly as a child," we are told, "and continued to do so episodically throughout her adult life." Carly Simon reputedly first began to sing because her mother used to tell her, when she stammered as a child, "Sing it!" Stutterers can also whisper without difficulty, read in unison or chant, or gain assistance from any kind of rhythm, because it helps them pattern their speech in time. Some also discover they can be fluent in a foreign language (like an uncle of Charles Darwin), or (like James Earl Jones) speak their lines without impediment onstage. Woody Allen, in *Broadway Danny Rose,* commented rather wittily on this whole phenomenon by portraying a ventriloquist who stuttered but whose dummy did not.

In their everyday lives, stutterers may also go to extraordinary lengths to avoid social interaction, such as adopting aliases, pretending they are deaf-mutes, or walking miles to an appointment rather than taking a cab. Philip Larkin recalled that up to the age of thirty or so he used to "hand over little slips of paper at the railway station saying third class to Birmingham, instead of actually trying to get it out." Others have been known to date only those whose names they think they can say, avoid buying houses on streets with names they think they can't, or choose vocations that don't require much talking, regardless of their other skills. "This stammer in my address," declares a character in Oliver Goldsmith's *She Stoops to Conquer* (1771), "can never permit me to soar above the reach of a milliner's apprentice." And indeed most careers have been affected in some way. Einer Boberg, currently Professor of Speech Pathology at the University of Alberta in Edmonton, Canada, recalls that in the summer of 1956, "I was a depressed young man who stuttered so severely that I had dropped out of school after Grade 9 because I could not face the testing in the local high school. After ploughing fields and shoveling manure for one year I mustered the courage to attend a church-sponsored High School where I could find refuge in quiet study, violin practice and singing in the choir."

Less conspicuously disabled was one state court judge who had managed by means of word substitution to disguise his stuttering from most of the outside world. When he was offered a federal judgeship, however, he declined, because, as he explained, "while I was allowed to paraphrase the charge to the jury in the state court, no such latitude in federal court was allowed. I would have had to read the charge word for word."

More pathetic is the story of the college dropout who took a clerical job but still "couldn't collect his paychecks because he was unable to say his name."

Stutterers are to be found, of course, in every walk of life.

And where celebrity or renown has been achieved, a tremendous if invisible struggle has often taken place behind the scenes. A list of well-known contemporaries is easy enough to draw up, and might include: John Updike, Edward Hoagland, Alfred Kazin, Harold Brodkey, and Robert Heinlein (among the writers); the singers Carly Simon and Mel Tillis; actors Austin Pendleton, Sam Neill, Jimmy Stewart, and James Earl Jones; John Russell, art critic of *The New York Times;* Clive Barnes, theater critic of the *New York Post;* Walter Wriston, the former chairman of Citicorp; dress designer Oscar de la Renta; Bob Love, former star of the Chicago Bulls; Lester Hayes, onetime star defensive cornerback for the Oakland Raiders; and so on.

But celebrity may claim no special dispensation here of praise. The perseverance of the everyday stutterer—unheralded and anonymous, with no laurels to encircle his brow—can be quite as heroic, in the face of constant frustration, humiliation, and defeat. At the end of Samuel Beckett's *Waiting for Godot,* there is a moment of dialogue that might be drawn from that life:

> ESTRAGON: I can't go on like this.
> VLADIMIR: That's what you think.

Not surprisingly, some stutterers will do just about anything to find relief. The odyssey of one took him through all the various therapy centers in the United States, then to Europe, where he stopped first at the shrine at Lourdes, where handicapped people have claimed miraculous cures. From Lourdes (uncured) he proceeded to Rome, where he visited a clinic in which stuttering children "were taught to paint and speak at the same time." In Vienna, he next encountered methods that emphasized relaxation, rhythmic breathing, and slow measured speech. In Munich, patients were encouraged to speak in a way that was "enthusiastic and full of melody and intonation." In Sweden, they were treated with tranquilizers and other neuroleptic drugs.

Others have tried weight lifting, prolonged silence, sighing, finger thumping, reading aloud with their teeth clenched, even "sitting around with a bib for a couple of days" (as one afflicted congressman recalls) "chewing carrots and making vocal sounds." When the interviewer, taken aback, asked him: "You just chewed carrots and talked for two days?" he replied, "Yes, chewed carrots and talked. And the carrot juice used to drip out of my mouth onto this big bib." In the tragic-comic/absurdist history of stuttering therapy, all such measures are but variations on cures that litter the historical stage.

# Part Two

*Conundrum*

# Chapter Three

Stuttering is probably as old as speech itself. Ancient Egyptian records allude to the disorder, and a fervent prayer to be delivered from it has been found on a cuneiform tablet from Mesopotamia, dating to 2500 B.C. In a slightly later papyrus from Egypt's Middle Kingdom stuttering is poignantly described as "to speak haltingly, as one who is sad." The disorder is also mentioned in a Chinese poem from the Han Dynasty, and at the biblical town of Beth Shemish a clay tablet has been unearthed on which may be read the anguished appeal, "O God! Cut through the backbone of my stuttering. Remove the spring of my impediment."

In Homer there is a term for speechlessness as a defect (not a transient emotional state), and in *Oedipus at Colonus* Sophocles uses a word meaning "privation of voice." The same word also occurs with the same meaning in Herodotus (born c. 484 B.C.) in connection with an anecdote about Croesus, the Lydian king. But in his anecdote about Battus, a Cretan born with a speech impediment, there is a more specific reference. Herodotus's phrase for his condition is *ischnophonos kai traulos,* which might best be translated as "a strained and stammering voice." Battus consulted the Oracle at Delphi about it, and the Oracle enigmatically replied that he should sail to Libya and there found a colony. He did so, at Cyrene, and (other commentators allege) his impediment disappeared. Perhaps the story is meant to suggest the therapeutic value of a change of scene. In any case, the Greek verb for stammering *(battarisdo)* derives from his name.

Aristotle in his discussion of speech anatomy in his treatise *On the History of Animals* also uses, in addition to *ischnophonos* and *traulos,* the word *psellos* to designate a speech defect involving "the omission of one particular letter or syllable." The word is onomatopoeic, and he may in fact have coined it to distinguish his own impediment, for he is said to have had a kind of stammer or lisp. Lisping he defined elsewhere (in his *Problems)* as an inability to master a letter, and "hesitancy" or stuttering as "the inability to join one letter to another with sufficient speed."

With regard to the latter, he asks, "Why is it that of all animals Man alone is apt to hesitate in his speech?" He concludes that it is because only man possesses reason, and cannot always "express his meaning continuously." This happens to children when they are learning to talk, to people who drink too much, and to others simply because they think faster than they can speak. But then there are those "melancholic" souls who "hesitate habitually." Aristotle was therefore careful to distinguish the malady itself from accidental instances of it. Yet he ultimately blamed the physical problem on the tongue, as moving too slowly "into position for uttering a second sound."

Aristotle's observations and conclusions dominated the discussion of stuttering and other speech disorders for the next fifteen hundred years. Indeed, it would long be assumed on his authority that the tongue was the chief organ of speech—even though there is no such thing, of course, since speech is a neurologically coordinated function of the entire organism. Nevertheless, language itself seemed almost to identify the two, since in numerous "tongues" (as we say), including Greek and Latin, the words for tongue and language are the same.

Following Aristotle, Hippocrates thought the impediment might arise from the speaker "thinking of fresh things before he has expressed what was already in his thoughts," but associated the condition in general with "aridity." His treatment (supposing the tongue to be engorged with black bile) was blistering.

Galen, the "Hippocrates of the Romans," as he was called (though a Greek, he lived under Roman rule), offered an anatomical analysis of speech that was considerably advanced. He understood and accurately described for the most part the operation of the larynx and the role of the articulators in modifying sounds, and rather beautifully and aptly described vocalization as expelled air striking an aulos or two-reeded flute. In one notable vivisection experiment, he also tied off the recurrent laryngeal nerve to show that the brain controls the voice. But he attributed stuttering specifically to an abnormality of the tongue—hypothesizing that, depending upon the case or age of the patient, it was either too short or too long, too wet or too dry. In most instances (following Hippocrates), he thought aridity was the cause, and to moisten the tongue sufficiently, prescribed wrapping it in little towels soaked in lettuce juice.

In the early Christian era, the Roman physician and philosopher Cornelius Celsus recommended gargling with concoctions of pennyroyal, hyssop, and thyme; chewing mustard, garlic, and onions (as stimulants); rubbing the tongue with lazerwort; and (to help relax the articulators) massaging the head, neck, mouth, and chin. As the therapeutic coup de grâce, the patient was "to immerse his head in cold water, eat horseradish, and vomit." Breathing exercises also had a place in his regimen, and regular exercise to strengthen the lungs. For those "tongue-tied from birth," however, "whose tongues are tied down to the part underlying it . . . in such cases the extremity of the tongue is to be seized with forceps, and the membrane under it stretched with a hook and cut, great care being taken not to injure the veins close by." Afterward, the mouth was to be rinsed with vinegar and water (an early antiseptic solution), and frankincense applied to the wound. He acknowledged, however, the uncertainty of the operation, and cited a case in which the tongue was "undercut so far that it could be protruded well beyond the teeth, yet the power of speech did not result."

Division of the frenum, as this procedure came to be called, recommended itself as a cure for stuttering because the frenum, a sublingual ligament attached to the tongue, was thought to restrain or "bridle" its movement. *Frenum* in Latin means "bridle," and the English phrase "unbridled tongue" originated as a pun on the Latin term. In its most primitive form, the procedure had been a folk remedy, for Galen mentions that "midwives used to cut away that membrane with their nails." With Celsus, it achieved official medical sanction.

In fact, from Celsus on, articulatory defects were generally attributed to the manner in which the sublingual ligaments connected the tongue to the jaw. Real or imagined abnormalities in their length or attachment were adduced to explain difficulties in pronouncing certain sounds, as in 1608, when the physician Fabricius Hildanus cut the frenum of his little brother because he supposed its unnatural thickness prevented the tongue from being raised to the palate or teeth.

Aside from frenectomy, speech pathology during the Middle Ages was based on the doctrine of the four humors, by which all general pathological conditions were explained. Although classical in origin, and accepted in principle by Hippocrates and Galen, it remained for Avicenna and other Islamic commentators to give it definitive form. This doctrine held

that human beings were a microcosm composed, like the macrocosm in which they lived and of which they were a part, of four basic elements—air, fire, earth, and water—and that these were in turn characterized by four qualities of heat, dryness, cold, and moisture. An individual's physical and mental attributes arose from and were determined by four chief fluids, called humors, in the body: blood, phlegm, yellow bile or choler, and black bile.

A person's characteristic nature and individual temperament were determined according to this doctrine by the relative proportions in his or her makeup of these four constituent and vital humors. The four classical temperaments or complexions which survive today as popular psychological types were sanguine, phlegmatic, choleric, and melancholic.

Bilious or choleric temperaments were hot and dry; sanguine (or "bloody"), hot and moist; phlegmatic, moist and cold; and melancholic, cold and dry. Any imbalance in the individual's normal proportions tended to disease. In the case of stuttering, "the actual disease was not the speech defect," as one scholar notes, "but the humoral imbalance affecting the whole organism." Each complexion therefore required a different approach; and it is for this reason (otherwise perplexing) that some physicians diagnosed the tongue as too wet, others as too dry. In effect, they were treating a different disease.

Nevertheless, at about the time of Celsus, it became axiomatic among physicians that humidity caused lingual paralysis (the moistness of a lisp seeming to confirm this), and that stuttering was the result of excessive humidity in the brain. Their task accordingly was to dry the patient out. To do this, they administered purgatives and astringent gargles, prescribed cauteries and blisters on the neck and behind the ears, and on occasion even encased the whole head in plaster to dry it out. To dessicate the tongue specifically, they rubbed it with salt, honey, and sage.

This was the therapy adopted by Rhazes, one of the greatest of Islamic physicians, who was born about A.D. 865 near Tehran. Sometimes called the "Galen to the Arabs," he acutely noted that stuttering tended to occur on initial sounds, and was perhaps the first to observe that it was more common among men.

Avicenna, his more famous and influential compatriot (born at Bukhara in A.D. 980), was also largely traditional, although he redefined stuttering as the inability to say a word "unless one or more of its component syllables are repeated several times." He also emphasized deep breathing for spasms of the epiglottis, and suggested an alternative procedure for surgery on the tongue. To avoid unnecessary bleeding and protect the sublingual veins, he recommended "that the membrane itself not be cut, but perforated towards the root with a needle, and tied. For this thread, if tightened daily, manipulates the membrane gently, and in a short time."

Other physicians made their own contributions down the line. John of Gaddesden, much esteemed by Chaucer and court physician to Edward III, gave some attention to stuttering, and prescribed for its relief a medicinal lozenge compacted primarily of castoreum (an antispasmodic), to be dissolved under the tongue. He also recommended gently rubbing the tongue with nasturtium juice. Division of the frenum, on the other hand, was the preferred procedure of Lanfranc of Milan, an Italian physician who fled to Lyons around 1270, and became "the founder of French surgery." He used a red-hot silver razor rather than a knife or thread. Bernard of Gordon, a lecturer in medicine at Montpellier in the early fourteenth century, was more interested in the language development of children. He noted that "there is a period in the lives of all children when they become 'nonfluent' and are unable to say what they want to say without stammering. This usually occurs between the ages of two and four when their speech is in the process of becoming more complex and their grammar and vocabulary more sophisticated." Bernard's observation could fit comfortably today into the most up-to-date textbook.

By the sixteenth century, the new anatomical research of Vesalius, Leonardo, and others prepared the way for a number of medical advances, but new treatments for stuttering did not result. The celebrated Italian physician, Hieronymus Mercurialis (1530–1606), speculated that stuttering might be aggravated by "deep thought," lack of sleep, and "immoderate Venus" (too much sex), but on the whole subscribed to the usual dessication procedures and a dietary regimen that favored spicy foods over nuts, pastry, and fish. On the other hand, if the tongue was deemed too dry, a savory concoction of marshmallow, water lily leaves, and sweet oil of almonds might be tried, as well as gargling with breast milk. Salves were also to be rubbed along the spine. In fact, there was nothing new in these prescriptions: they were borrowed almost verbatim from a tenth-century Persian physician, Ali ibn al Abbas.

In his *Treatise on the Diseases of Children* published in 1583, however, Mercurialis proved more advanced. Beyond the insights of Bernard of Gordon cited above, he pointed out that children should not be treated for stuttering until they were at least seven years old, "since before that time it cannot be known whether their speech is defective or not . . . because it often happens that children stutter up until their sixth or seventh year, and are nonetheless spontaneously cured; on account of which, once it is certain that a spontaneous end is not to be put to the disease, treatment must be entered into immediately." Surgery might be required (by Avicenna's method), or purgatives compacted of agaric and cloves to be administered in the form of pills. "That these may be swallowed the more easily by children," he adds, "they may be hidden in a little cake, or some jam." Nosedrops combining beetroot and betony juice mixed with coriander were also to be given to help dehumidify the brain.

Although the "Western tradition," as it is sometimes called, was more advanced in this field than elsewhere, some acknowledgment should be made of the speech pathology of ancient India. Ancient Sanskrit scholars had a relatively sound understanding of speech and language development; and an empirical knowledge of vocal anatomy: not inappropriately, the larynx with its vocal cords was compared to a stringed instrument. Some speech and language disorders were thought to be congenital (due to ungratified cravings of the mother during pregnancy), while others were ascribed to meteorological conditions, diet, or trauma. In the treatment of stuttering, tongue exercises were standard, and their typical herbal adjunct included clarified butter, eggplant seeds mixed with honey, and cumin and whin seeds mixed with salt. Sour fruit was recommended to stimulate the tongue and dissolve excessive phlegm.

Expert treatises, of course, are not the only source of useful information (even on technical subjects), and just as Alan Dugan's magnificent poem on stuttering, quoted toward the beginning of this book, generally reflected the understanding (and "sound advice of experts") at the time it was composed, so allusions to stuttering in the culture and literature of the Renaissance afford a broader appreciation of what was thought or known.

Perhaps the lowest common denominator could be found in the commedia dell'arte or popular comic theater of Renaissance Italy, where one of the stock, or masked, characters was called Tartaglia ("the Stammerer"). Almost invariably this character was an object of ridicule, but the label was in fact generic—anyone with indistinct articulation might be so described. In this way, for example, Niccolò Fontana (Tartaglia), the Venetian mathematician who discovered a method for solving cubic equations and originated the science of ballistics, acquired his name. During a French assault on Brescia (a Venetian possession) in 1512, his jaws and palate were cleft by a saber. He was thirteen years old at the time, and thereafter spoke with difficulty (though not with a stammer). He was nicknamed Tartaglia anyway, and defiantly adopted it as his surname as a man.

On the other hand, it is more edifying to discover that fourteen years before Mercurialis was born (and sixty-seven years before he published his great treatise on childhood diseases), a basic understanding of childhood speech development had evidently been grasped. At least as early as 1516 (but perhaps as early as 1440 when it may have been composed), we may read in a *Lyfe of Seynt Birgette* that she already stood out as a little girl because "shee spake complete and full wordes, nat stuttyne lyke the maner of other children that begynne to speke." Moreover, it was generally realized that for therapy to be effective the disorder had to be dealt with early, especially if inborn. Thus one Andrew Boorde, in *A Breviary of Healthe* (1547), wrote: "Whan Stuttynge . . . doth come by nature, it cannot be holpen except it be reformed in youth by some discrete tutor."

Specific manifestations of the disorder were also detailed. In a sermon delivered in 1574, the Swiss theologian John Calvin spoke of a man who stuttered so badly that he could not "draw forth one onely woord." He was referring, of course, to complete blocking. More interesting is a passage in *As You Like It* in which Shakespeare, who had obviously noticed that stutterers tend either to hurry their words (out of fear of blocking) or to block, compares their speech to pouring wine from a bottle with a long neck:

I pr'ythee, tell me, who is it? quickly, and speak apace. I would thou could'st stammer, that thou might'st pour this

concealed man out of thy mouth, as wine comes out of a
narrow mouthd bottle, either too much at once, or none at
all.

At about the same time, the great English composer
William Byrd recommended singing as a "singular good
remedie for stutting and stammering," since speech, as exemplified by song, must be rhythmically patterned in time. No
one, however, was more thorough in his observations than
Sir Francis Bacon in his *Sylva Sylvarum,* published in 1627:

> Divers, we see, doe Stut. The Cause may bee, (in most) the
> Refrigeration of the Tongue; Whereby it is lesse apt to move,
> And, therefore, wee see that Naturalls doe generally Stut:
> And wee see in those that Stut, if they drinke Wine moder-
> ately, they Stut, less, because it heateth: And so we see that
> they that stut doe Stut more in the first offer to speake, than
> in Continuance; Because the Tongue is, by Motion some-
> what heated. In some also, it may be (though rarely) the Dri-
> nesse of the Tongue; which likewise maketh it lesse apt to
> move, as well as Cold; For it is an Affect that it cometh to
> some Wise and Great Men; as it did unto Moses, who was
> *Linguae Praepeditae* [of tangled tongue]; And many Stutters
> we finde are very Cholericke Men; Choler Enducing a Dri-
> nesse in the tongue.

To paraphrase, he tells us that stuttering affects a wide variety of people; that it cannot be taken as a sign of inferiority
(witness Moses); that drink sometimes helps (not by heat, as
he supposes, but as a relaxant); that it helps to warm up the
vocal apparatus before attempting to speak (which is true);
and that people who stutter usually have particular trouble
with initial sounds. I might add that Bacon's "Naturalls" are

Mercurialis's *Balbuties Naturales* (those who stutter because of a natural or humoral imbalance), as distinguished from *Balbuties Accidentales* (those who stutter due to sudden emotions or injury). And when he mentions "Refrigeration" and "Drinesse" of the tongue as alternative causes, he is referring to the cold/dry qualities of which the melancholic temperament is made up.

Finally, his remark that "many Stutters we finde are Cholericke Men" is also meant in the "temperamental" sense. Although some people may stutter less when angered (Updike in his *Memoirs* remarks this about himself), the colloquial connection between the two has long been commonplace, in part because even normal speakers may sputter (in a way that resembles stuttering) when so aroused. "It is a worlde to here hym stammer when he is angryd," wrote Jehan Palsgrave in 1530; and in Ben Jonson's *Poetaster* (1601) a character exclaims: "Hee lookes bigge and begins to stut, for anger."

Another popular notion—that stuttering could be acquired by imitation—had yet to turn up in the treatises of physicians, but was already widespread. "If it [stuttering] do come with being in the company of a stutter or stamerer," advised Andrew Boorde in 1547, then (he said) associate with someone else. A century later Ben Jonson in his *Discoveries* (1640) wrote that some "Children . . . imitate the vices of stammerers so long, till at last they become such." And the seventeenth-century English scientist Robert Boyle was sure he had acquired his own impediment that way. These three (and doubtless others) clearly anticipated the Swiss physician Johann Amman, who is usually credited with being the first to suggest (in 1702) that stuttering was learned behavior—

"the contraction of a vicious habit which in time becomes inveterate."

In short, by the middle of the seventeenth century, most of the observable peculiarities of stuttering had been noted, and one or two new ideas had arisen as to its cause. But the only new treatment (an unpalatable one at that) was proposed by Johann Gottfried Hahn, a German, who thought the problem had to do with the hyoid bone. This small, U-shaped bone is situated deep in the muscles at the back of the tongue where it is suspended by ligaments from the base of the skull. Giovanni Battista Morgagni (1682–1771), the founder of pathological anatomy, also supposed this bone was the culprit; but neither could say exactly what the problem was. And Hahn, a bit rashly, suggested the bone be cut out. This could only have had the most unfortunate results, since its ascertainable function is to provide an anchor point for the muscles of the tongue and for those in the upper part of the front of the neck.

Our understanding of the history of stuttering is immeasurably broadened by attention to biography. The number of stutterers who have achieved renown is imposing, and it is natural enough to be curious about the impact of the defect on their lives. For the moralization of our curiosity we might (though with some misgiving) turn to the words of one of the afflicted, W. Somerset Maugham: "I do not believe they are right who say that the defects of famous men should be ignored. I think it is better that we should know them. Then, though we are conscious of having faults as glaring as theirs, we can believe that that is no hindrance to our achieving also something of their virtues." Maugham is not quite right, of course: the obvious hindrance would be lack of greatness in ourselves. Nor is stuttering a "fault" in the colloquial sense. The better and more universal moral may be drawn from a couplet by Robert Herrick:

> Fortune did never favour one
> Fully, without exception.

Herrick's moral applies in extremis to Aesop (c. 550 B.C.), whose semilegendary life would give hope to anyone thinking himself ill-favored by the gods. Born a slave, he was "of all other men most defformed," we are told, "and evyll shapen. For he had a greate heade, large visage, longe jawes, sharpe eyen, a shorte necke, crooked backe, greate belly, greate legges, and large fete. And that which was worse, he coulde not speke."

One day, laboring in his master's fields, he sought refuge from the sun and fell asleep in the shade of a tree. The Goddess of Hospitality appeared to him in a dream and gave him "sapyence and abylite" and the gift of speech "without empesshement [impediment]." As a result, his "singular wytte" soon became apparent, and his whole life changed. He became a master storyteller, famed for his animal fables, a solver of riddles, and "subtill in cavillacions," all of which drew him to the attention of the Babylonian court. He rose from slave to royal advisor, only to lose his life in the end at the hands of Babylonian subjects grown jealous of his power.

Of far mightier (but still semilegendary renown) is the biblical prophet Moses, who after Yahweh spoke to him from the Burning Bush and called for him to deliver the Hebrews from Egypt, protested his unworthiness, and begged to be released from his task. Yahweh pledged signs and miracles to confirm his authority, but Moses replied (Exodus 4:1,10): "They will not believe me, nor hearken unto my voice. . . . I am not eloquent, neither heretofore, nor since thou hast spoken unto thy servant: but I am slow of speech and of a slow tongue." Both Hebrew and Christian scholars agree that these biblical phrases refer to stuttering. Down through the ages rabbinical tales, Christian sermons, and secular literature alike have identified his impediment as such, and by the Renaissance "stammering" and "stuttering" were regular epithets attached to his name. Bacon's Latin phrase ("of tangled tongue"), however, also suggests a familiarity with the Koran, in which the impediment of Moses is more explicitly evoked:

> "Lord, open my breast," said Moses,
> "and do Thou ease for me my task,
> Unloose the knot upon my tongue,
> that they may understand my words."

Circumstantial evidence helps to confirm the diagnosis, for Moses exhibited classic avoidance behavior when he insisted that his brother Aaron speak for him. An impatient (but finally understanding) Yahweh agrees (Exodus 4:16): "And he shall be thy spokesman unto the people and he shall be to thee instead of a mouth."

In classical antiquity, the Roman poet Vergil reportedly stuttered, but his early biographers are as vague about his impediment as Aristotle's are about his lisp. The Greek orator Demosthenes (the very first person in the history of the world, as Werner Jaeger noted, about whom we have any concrete biographical information) is another matter, and possibly the most famous stutterer who ever lived. Almost every schoolboy knows (or used to know) something of his story, and any number of stutterers down through the ages have emulated aspects of his self-begotten cure.

Generally regarded as the greatest orator of ancient times, Demosthenes was born in Athens, Greece, in 384 B.C. His father, a wealthy sword-maker and cabinet manufacturer, died when he was seven, and Demosthenes grew up in reduced circumstances in the care of his mother. It may be that, over-protective of his delicate constitution, she mothered him too much, for she refused to allow him to take part in the gymnastic exercises that were important to the education of every Athenian youth. As a result, he spent a somewhat sheltered and solitary adolescence prematurely immersed in books. When he came of age, he stood to gain a considerable inheritance, but the guardians appointed to safeguard it cheated him out of most of the estate. He brought suit against them, and notwithstanding his stutter, argued his own case in court. After many adjournments and appeals, he ultimately prevailed, but was unable to recover more than the exiguous remains.

The experience, however, whetted his appetite for debate and he embarked at once upon a career in public life. He studied the works of the oratorical masters (Isocrates and others), but his early rhetorical manner was rough. Sometimes he mumbled, at other times he spoke in disconnected bursts, or was led by his impediment into confused and rambling asides. The first Athenian crowds he ventured to address laughed at him, and after one such rebuff, a friend and well-known actor took him aside and began to work with him on his speech. Together they recited passages from the works of the great dramatists (in particular, Sophocles and

Euripides), and in this way he came to understand more clearly the importance of coordinating his voice and gestures with his words. However, elocution lessons could take him only so far; and in order to achieve true flexibility in his delivery, he had to conquer his impediment, which stood so intractably in his way.

He saw what he must do. To clarify his pronunciation (he had particular trouble with the letter "r"), he practiced speaking with pebbles under his tongue, and to strengthen his voice, stood on the shore of the sea and declaimed above the roar of the waves. To develop more powerful lungs, he strapped lead weights to his chest and recited to himself as he ran uphill. He also built for himself an underground study to which he used to retire to practice for months at a time. To prevent himself from going outside, he made himself grotesque by shaving his head and beard completely on one side. He also set up a full-length mirror in which to study and correct his gestures, and went so far as to suspend a razor-sharp sword above one shoulder to check its disagreeable shrugs.

Nor during all this time did he neglect the literary aspects of the orator's art. Aside from his study of the masters, he copied out Thucydides's long history of the Peloponnesian War eight times in order to improve his command of the Greek language (which it exemplified at its best) and to absorb the historical lessons of the text. After he emerged from seclusion, it became his daily habit to review each night conversations and speeches he had heard that day, and to imagine rebuttals to them or ways in which their delivery might have been improved.

The therapeutic regimen Demosthenes imposed upon himself was fanatical, and the austere firmness and determination it required indelibly marked his face. For in all the surviving busts of him he seems never to unbend his stern and imposing brow. Some of the busts, not incidentally, show the lower lip raised against the gum, an articulatory posture stutterers sometimes assume when struggling with a sound.

For a time, Demosthenes wrote speeches for others; then at the age of thirty, he made his official debut. The Athenian Assembly (a completely democratic body) had gathered to consider what to do about a rumored threat from Persia. Demosthenes stood up and, in a tightly reasoned speech, urged the city to rebuild its navy while trying to defuse the crisis by diplomatic means. He also seized the occasion to outline a plausible new tax policy that would enable the city to finance his rearmament plans. "From that moment on," it is said, "Demosthenes' career was virtually the history of Athenian foreign policy."

In subsequent years, as leader of the Athenian democratic party (which placed him in opposition to the oligarchical aspirations of the rich), he roused Athens against Macedonian imperial ambitions, as incarnated first in the conquests of Philip of Macedon, then of Philip's son, Alexander the Great. Over the course of twenty-nine years, the rhetorical exhortations of Demosthenes were repeatedly required to steel the people's will.

In public forums, he seldom faltered, but in his everyday speech he was subject to constant relapse; and once, when sent to negotiate with Philip, he briefly lost control and stuttered so badly that his enemies in Athens never let him live it down.

As a result of complex political maneuvering, Demosthenes eventually found himself disgraced, condemned by the citizenry he had done so much to save. After the Greeks suffered defeat at the hands of the Macedonians, he committed suicide in 322 B.C.

Posterity made amends. After his death, the Athenians erected a bronze statue to his memory, and his speeches became the foundation of oratorical training in Roman schools. During the Middle Ages and the Renaissance, "his name was synonymous with eloquence." Queen Elizabeth I of England studied his orations in the original (with the help of the scholar Roger Ascham), and her own rhetorical felicities perhaps owed something to her admiration for his. Today, few names remain as gloriously familiar from the classical past.

That cannot be said, of course, of the Roman emperor Claudius, often portrayed as a dithering fool whose inept administration contributed to the decline of the empire. In recent years he has undergone something of a positive reassessment, but the ancient judgment was mixed. The Stoic philosopher Seneca, for example, cruelly ridiculed his infirmities in the *Pumpkinification of Claudius the God,* and Tacitus in his *Annals* depicted him as weak, incompetent, and oblivious to the corruption and debauchery of his court. Suetonius, in his brief biography, was equally harsh. On the other hand, he emerges from the works of Flavius Josephus, a contemporary Jewish historian, as a more ambiguous figure, and Cassius Dio's representation of him as an industrious, public-spirited ruler helped to correct the caricature. Pliny in his *Natural History* more influentially praised him as a master builder and patron of the arts, and most of the lesser-known Roman historians credit him with character and judgment above his faults.

Born Tiberius Claudius Drusus in Lugdunum (modern-day Lyons) on August 1, 10 B.C., Claudius's beginnings were both blessed and cursed. On the one hand, his father was the Roman governor of Gaul and the stepson of Augustus; his mother, the daughter of Marc Antony. With such a pedigree, he was the automatic recipient of wealth and power. However, he was also a sickly child, with multiple ills that have been variously ascribed to hydrocephalus, epilepsy, or a form of infantile paralysis associated with premature birth. His own mother complained that he was "unfinished by nature," and his stutter, nervous tremors, tics, and other infirmities persuaded his family that he was mentally deficient and (as he grew to manhood) "incapable of acting with that dignity expected of a prince of the house." Suetonius says that he staggered when he walked, nervously tossed his head from side to side, laughed uncontrollably when merry, or (when enraged) "slobbered horribly at the mouth." Augustus, fearing that he would make himself ridiculous at social functions, made sure he always had an escort; and at one point subjected him to the supervision of a muleteer with the idea that brute discipline might help him shape up.

Claudius remained unreconstructed; yet gradually his capacities also made themselves known. He demonstrated intellectual curiosity by his diligent study of history (encouraged by the historian Livy), and in time Augustus himself began to notice that "in important matters, where his mind does not wander, the nobility of his character can be seen." In public presentations, he learned to declaim without always stammering (even though his conversation remained "unclear"), and in A.D. 41, when he was unexpectedly enthroned, he proved worthy of his elevation and of the role destiny had assigned.

As emperor, he extended Roman rule in North Africa, made Britain a province of the empire, and in his domestic policies seemed to appreciate that the welfare of the people reposed in his care. Though he expelled the Jews from Rome during one troubled juncture of his reign, elsewhere he confirmed Jewish rights and privileges, and in Alexandria tried to protect the Jews without provoking Egyptian nationalism. In a surviving letter addressed to that city, he asked Jews and non-Jews alike to relinquish their "obstinate mutual enmity," which could only prove destructive to them both.

The apparent discrepancy between his early lack of promise and the accomplishments of his rule lends credence to a tradition, inadvertently begun by Suetonius and developed most recently in a pair of historical novels by Robert Graves, that Claudius had deliberately exaggerated his own infirmities in order to appear negligible to those ruthlessly striving for power. "His health," Suetonius wryly reminds us, "was wretched until he succeeded to the throne, when it suddenly became excellent."

But all his shrewdness could not save him in the end. In October A.D. 54, he was poisoned by his second wife, Agrippina, in a plot to advance her own son, Nero, to the throne.

Sovereigns tend to die hard, and so from Claudius to England's Charles I we may scarcely break our stride. Born on November 19, 1600, to James I, Queen Elizabeth's successor, he was (like Claudius) a sickly child, slow to learn how to walk or talk, much fretted over by apothecaries, and the cause of much royal exasperation and concern. After advertisement was made for a governess, many great ladies, we are told, "came to see the boy with the hope of being granted the influential position of his care." However, "when they did see how weake a child he was, and not likely to live, their hearts were downe, and none of them was desirous to take charge of him." King James decided to clip his frenum (according to "the sound advice of experts" at the time) and to put him in iron boots to strengthen his ankles and legs. Fortunately, Lady Carey, in whose care he was eventually placed, tactfully opposed such remedies, and under her more patient coaxing, the health of the young prince bloomed. With the help of a rocking horse and a little propelling chair with wheels, he soon grew sturdy, and although his stuttered speech came very slowly, he showed a substantial aptitude for languages, and under successive tutors learned Greek and Latin, Italian and French.

He also worked hard to become athletic, in part to compensate for his diminutive height. He developed into an excellent shot, rode well, took part in jousts, and was good at tennis and golf. Indeed, everyone remarked upon his determination to overcome his handicaps, and it was noted that even as an infant his strong spirit had impressed the royal astrologer Lilly, who predicted he would prove "very wilful and obstinate" as an adult.

Charles's shyness and reserve, however, were abiding, and he stammered throughout his life. In emulation of Demosthenes, he practiced speaking with pebbles under his tongue; tried singing (which he found helpful); but in the end found it most effective to form each sentence carefully in his mind before attempting to speak. After his older brother, Henry, the heir apparent, died suddenly in 1612, Charles applied himself with even greater determination so as to be worthy to take his place. In 1616 he was created Prince of Wales, and when he appeared in that role in public for the first time, a contemporary could state that there was "nothing undignified about him"—even if, though an otherwise dashing prince, he "looked rather sad, dispirited, and remote."

Without rehearsing the events that led to England's Civil

War, it is unfortunately the case that his inability to communicate directly with Parliament (due to his stammer) probably had an unfavorable influence on his affairs. At least, a number of his friends thought so and traced the origins of the schism to his first speech from the throne. This he awkwardly concluded by saying, "Because I am unfit for much speaking, I mean . . . to have my Lord-Keeper speak for me in most things," just as Moses had Aaron serve as his mouth. In conversation and in council, he tended to be rather brief (some thought surly), but a contemporary assures us that "he had a quicker perception and did sooner understand a case" than any of his ministers. And in 1631, the Spanish ambassador noted that the king "gave audience easily . . . listened with attention and answered to the point."

During the long Civil War, Charles occasionally demonstrated a kind of pithy eloquence, and after his capture proved "very majestic and steady," according to his friend, Sir Philip Warwick, "and was never discomposed in mind." At his trial, he conducted his own defense with masterful skill, and to the mystification and amazement of all those attending, throughout the ordeal—even to the end of his scaffold confession—"he stammered nothing at all but spoke very distinctly with much courage and magnanimity."

One of the king's most gifted subjects, born about the time he ascended the throne, was the chemist and natural philosopher Robert Boyle. Boyle stuttered acutely, and became convinced he had "contracted" the affliction as a child by imitating the "stuttering Habitude" of a playmate his own age. He religiously interpreted his misery as perhaps "a just judgment upon my Derision, turning the effects of God's Anger into the Matter of my Sport." Over the years, he tried choral singing and other therapies (to little avail), and the moral he derived from his condition was: "So Contagious & catching are men's Faults . . . that by being imitated but in jest, come to be learn'd (& acquir'd) in earnest."

Boyle was a bit of a hypochondriac, and throughout his life fussed about his health. He was scrupulously abstemious in his diet, and at the slightest change in the weather immediately adjusted his clothes. He also tried to spare his mind all contamination of frivolity. He scorned light reading of any kind, and "to fix his volatile fancy and . . . curb the roving wildness of his wandering thoughts," concentrated at idle moments on mathematical problems, especially the abstraction of square and cube roots. He mastered Latin, Greek, French, and German, took up Hebrew under the instruction of a rabbi when he was sixty years old, and along the way learned to control his stutter by developing a slow and deliberate style of speech. According to the diarist John Evelyn, once Boyle was able to struggle past an initial sound "he proceeded without the least interruption in his discourse."

Although his somewhat humorless demeanor incited the satire of Swift, who also caricatured Boyle's literary style (in "A Meditation upon a Broom-Stick"), Boyle's knowledge of many subjects was truly vast. His contributions to chemistry (in particular his experiments on the properties of gases), and his corpuscular view of matter (which anticipated the modern theory of chemical elements), earned him lasting renown.

Boyle's approach to his stutter may have benefited from his correspondence with Cotton Mather, the greatest of New England's Puritan divines. Born in Boston in 1663, the son and grandson of illustrious Congregational ministers, Mather decided at a very early age to devote his life to study and prayer. By eleven he was competent at Latin, Greek, and

Hebrew; was admitted to Harvard at age twelve; delivered his first sermon at sixteen; and two years later was offered his own congregation and church.

Although he believed in witchcraft (for which he has often been excoriated), Mather's learned and enlightened interests were even more eclectic than Boyle's. Nothing seems to have escaped his attention. One contemporary scholar, who knew him well, exclaimed: " 'Tis almost amazing how much He had read & studied—How much He had wrote and published—How much He corresponded abroad . . . How many Languages, Histories, Arts, and Sciences, both ancient and modern He was familiarly versed in—What a vast Amassment of Learning He had grasp'd in his Mind, from all sorts of Writings." Mather's private library was by far the largest in New England, and even light reading (which indeed distinguished him from Boyle) formed part of his occasional fare. While he had no patience for frivolity, he also stressed (in his advice to budding ministers) that a scholar should not be "an Odd, Starv'd, Lank sort of thing, who had lived only on Hebrew Roots all his Days." His own work encompassed more than four hundred volumes, and included, aside from sermons and theological tracts, works of history, biography, fable, and poetry, manuals of practical piety, and essays on scientific and medical topics of the day. He ably expounded a germ theory of disease, discoursed on magnetism, and in response to an account of his own pioneering efforts to introduce smallpox inoculation to New England, was elected to the Royal Society of London. Mather also wrote the first treatise on stuttering in America, which appears as a chapter in *The Angel of Bethesda,* a collection of medical essays written toward the end of his life. Speaking as if about another (but transparently about himself), he wrote: "I know of one who had been very much a Stammerer, and no words can tell, how much his Infirmity did Encumber and Embitter the first years of his Pilgrimage." He recalled the continual "Pain how to get thro' the Speaking Part" of every human encounter, the "Inhumane Derision" of others in response to his faltering, and the "Thousands of Supplications for a Free Speech" he had poured out to Christ.

Not unlike Boyle, but more gravely, Mather discerned in his impediment the hand of a chastening God. In his youth, it had persisted despite his father's devout fasting and his own numerous prayers, and because it threatened to keep him from the pulpit—"a Thing as much despaired of, as anything in the World"—he had even regarded it for a time as a sign that he was damned. Upon the advice of a wise and sympathetic schoolmaster (Elijah Corlet), however, who visited him at Harvard, he eventually learned "to oblige himself to a dilated Deliberation" in his speech, which involved a kind of "drawling . . . little short of Singing," that at the same time allowed him to more carefully consider his words. To illustrate his method, Corlet had recited a verse from Homer, slowly prolonging each syllable, and then explained: "By this Deliberation, the Organs of Your Speech will be so Habituated unto Right-Speaking, that you will by Degrees, and Sooner than you imagine, grow Able to speak as fast again, as you did . . . Tho' my advice is, Beware of Speaking too fast, as long as you Live."

As long as Mather lived, Corlet's method helped him, despite occasional relapses severe enough at times "to threaten . . . to render me unserviceable." Although he remained convinced that (in his own case) the sins of Anger and Pride had something to do with his chastisement (which led him to constantly reexamine his life), he did not neglect the coordinate possibility of a neurological cause. "The Original of this Infirmity," he perspicaciously wrote in 1724, "may be a Weaknesse upon that pair of Nerves, which give Motion and Vigour to the Organs of Speech." And his reflections on the matter (as might be hoped for from a man who inhabited both worlds) form something of a bridge between the old science and the new.

# Chapter Four

In the seventeenth century language was still widely regarded as a gift from God; in the eighteenth century it was
primarily understood as a physiologic mechanism. With
Morgagni, the humoral theory began to be replaced by an
idea of the human body as a complex machinery of inter-
related parts, or systems of parts, working harmoniously
together. In the field of language study, there arose a corresponding preoccupation with mechanical models of speech,
which led to various attempts to construct speaking machines.
At the end of the century, one such machine—a pneumo-
mechanical device for the production of artificial speech
sounds—was built by Wilhelm von Kempelen, an Austrian
phonetician, who hoped that it might be used to help cure
"some of those persons who have a defective pronunciation."

In keeping with the new perspective, remedial approaches toward stuttering emphasized elocution exercises, clear and correct articulation, and beating time when reading aloud. Since stutterers are able to sing because (it was not incorrectly thought) "the melody dictates to them the rhythm they are to use," rhythmic practice in declamation was adopted to help them get a feel for "the rhythmical pulsation . . . befitting their words."

The mechanism of the voice was also more precisely understood, not as a stringed or as a wind instrument, but as a combination of both: the vocal cords (or strings) being made to vibrate by air produce a sound modified by the articulators (like the stops on a flute).

Two outstanding eighteenth-century thinkers—both stammerers themselves—also psychologized the problem in new ways. One was Moses Mendelssohn (grandfather of the composer Felix), the other Erasmus Darwin (grandfather of the biologist).

Born in 1729, the son of an impoverished scribe of Dessau, Mendelssohn was so assiduously studious as a youth that by age fourteen he had become permanently hunched from bending over the Talmud and the works of Maimonides. In 1743 he moved to Berlin, where he became a silk merchant; but his commercial dealings always remained secondary to his intellectual pursuits. He became the friend and confidant of the dramatist Gotthold Lessing, a leading figure in the German Enlightenment; wrote on Leibniz, Spinoza, Plato, and others; engaged (reluctantly) in theological disputes, and translated the Psalms. An accomplished linguist, he knew Polish, French, and English as well as German and Hebrew, and by virtue of his learning and wisdom was christened the "German Socrates." But above all else he was committed to the acculturation of the German-Jewish community to German life. The Swiss theologian Johann Kaspar Lavater once paid tribute to him as "a companionable, brilliant soul, with pleasing ideas; the body of an Aesop; a man of keen insight, exquisite taste and erudition. He is a great venerator of all thinking minds and himself a metaphysician; an impartial judge of all works of taste; frank and openhearted in intercourse, more modest in his speech than in his writings, unaffected by praise. . . ."

It was Mendelssohn's speculation that stuttering was due to "a collision between many ideas, flowing simultaneously from the brain." This was a bit different from the Aristotelian hypothesis that a stutterer's tongue was too sluggish to keep pace with his thought. In Berlin, he joined an intellectual circle whose members occasionally read mathematical or philosophical papers to one another, but his stutter was unmanageable enough for him invariably to ask another member to read his paper aloud. With some poetic amusement, he once summed up his defects for his learned friends:

> Great you call Demosthenes,
> Stuttering orator of Greece;
> Hunchbacked Aesop you deem wise;—
> In your circle I surmise
> I am doubly wise and great.
> What in each was separate
> You in me united find,—
> Hump and heavy tongue combined.

This clever verse is made cleverer still by its submerged allusion to Moses, who (because of his "heavy tongue") had also asked others to speak for him, and for whom Mendelssohn, of course, was named.

As might be expected of a man whom Christian theologians made it their mission to convert, Mendelssohn did his best to avoid controversy, but sometimes utterly failed. One morning he awoke to discover that he had almost precipitated a pogrom in Prussia by criticizing the poems of Frederick the Great.

The responsibilities of being the most prominent Jew in Germany were not easy to bear.

By contrast, there probably never lived a more robustly cheerful, even carefree stutterer than Erasmus Darwin (1731–1802), the English physician and naturalist.

Educated in the classics, mathematics, and medicine at the universities of Cambridge and Edinburgh, Darwin opened a successful medical practice in Lichfield, England, in 1756, and in time acquired such a substantial name for himself that King George III offered to make him his personal physician. Darwin, however, preferred to remain in his country seat, where he could more easily indulge his manifold pursuits. He corresponded with Rousseau, Benjamin Franklin, and other prominent thinkers, was a founder of the Lunar Society of Birmingham, "the chief intellectual driving force behind the Industrial Revolution in England," and shared ideas with Matthew Boulton, James Watt, and Josiah Wedgwood, who did much to bring that revolution about. Darwin himself produced a number of working inventions, including designs for canal lifts, rotary pumps, horizontal windmills, flush toilets, and precursors of the rocket motor and the submarine. When not attending to his medical rounds, he also wrote several large treatises in verse, including *The Botanic Garden,* a long poem on horticultural themes; *Zoonomia, or The Laws of Organic Life,* a voluminous discussion of biological evolution, selective breeding, and the inheritance of mutations; and *Phytologia, or The Philosophy of Agriculture and Gardening,* a grand survey of vegetable life "and all that sustains it, from carbon dioxide down to manures." Embedded in these works was often new information; for example, he was the first to identify nitrogen and phosphorus as essential plant nutrients, and offered the most complete account of photosynthesis up until that time. In another long poem, *The Temple of Venus* (published posthumously), he traced in often dazzling couplets the evolution of life from microscopic organisms to Man. Indeed, without too much qualification it can be said that his grandson's ideas on heredity, adaptation, and natural selection were partially anticipated (and to some degree stimulated) by Erasmus's work. The English Romantic poets were also influenced by him, and Mary Shelley's *Frankenstein* owes its genesis to a discussion Byron and Shelley had about his ideas on the generation of life.

Darwin "stammered extremely," in the words of one contemporary, and "the closest attention was necessary in order to understand what he said." Nevertheless, Darwin himself believed his impediment had actually helped him (simply by attracting notice) when he was first starting out as a doctor, and he seems to have had a gift (which his stammer did not appreciably impede) for explaining any difficult subject with concision and wit. He was not a good man to quarrel with either, for when challenged in an argument, he "always revenged it by sarcasm of very keen edge."

In addition to stuttering, Darwin was stoop-shouldered, had a pockmarked face, and was hugely fat—in fact, a gap had to be cut into the side of his dining room table to accommodate his girth. Nevertheless, women were drawn to him, and he led a lusty life. He had twelve legitimate and illegitimate children, and at the age of fifty won out over several more dashing rivals for the hand of a beautiful widow of thirty-three. His own translation of an epigram by Martial might almost serve as the motto of his life:

> Wine, women, warmth, against our lives combine,
> But what is life without warmth, women, wine.

Much of his scientific writing was surprisingly erotic. Sexual allusions, for example, permeate *The Botanic Garden,* an encyclopedic work originally intended to lure readers through poetry to science by the versification of Linnaean botany. However, in the course of two thousand or so rhyming couplets, it developed into a highly romantic and anthropomorphic account of the sex life of plants. This included by analogy (for such is Nature's profusion) promiscuity and group sex. More generally, Darwin believed that an aesthetic sensibility could be traced "to the pleasure of the first nourishment derived from the soft and gently rounded maternal breast." In our maturer years, he wrote, "when any object of vision is presented to us, which by its waving or spiral lines bears any similitude to the female bosom . . . we feel a general glow of delight."

Darwin's appetite for life was ravenous, and the carriage he rode around in resembled a studio apartment. On one side were stacks of books that completely blocked the door; on the other, a hamper crammed with fruits, sweetmeats, cheese, and clotted cream. Rather conveniently, he believed that "eating an almost immeasurable abundance of sweet things" was good for his health. Nevertheless, he generally abstained from wine, in part because he was tempted to drink too much. This may have been because, as one anecdote suggests, it helped his speech. On a boating trip with some friends near Nottingham, for example, he got into a "high state of vinous exhilaration," and to the astonishment of his companions, suddenly stepped from the boat into the river and swam to shore. He emerged onto the bank, walked "coolly over the meadows towards the town," and when his friends finally caught up with him, found him in the marketplace holding forth to a crowd "without a trace of his usual stammer" from on top of a tub.

Darwin psychologized his own impediment as a kind of approach-avoidance conflict. Wanting to speak well, the stutterer is beset by a "corresponding fear of failure so great that the associations of the muscular motions of articulation become impaired." He then attempts in vain to regain control and a stuttering block, often accompanied by "various distortions of countenance," results. The more he tries willfully to correct the (normally automatic) "muscular associations," the more they "become dissevered by this greater exertion."

Darwin's therapeutic advice was not to try so hard to be articulate (or to make an impression, since he thought—extrapolating from himself—that it had to do with vanity), and at the same time to patiently correct the stuttered sounds:

> The art of curing this defect is to cause the stammerer to repeat the word, which he finds difficult to speak, eight or ten times with the initial letter, in a strong voice, or with an aspirate before it, as arable or harable; and at length to speak it softly with the initial letter P, parable. This should be practiced for weeks or months upon every word, which the stammerer hesitates in pronouncing. To this should be added much commerce with mankind, in order to acquire a carelessness about the opinions of others.

Modern speech pathologists will recognize in this passage foreshadowings of their own techniques of self-correction (repeating the word), gentle onset (beginning the word softly), and toughening exercises to help in the transference to social situations of newly acquired speech skills.

Darwin's own therapy was far ahead of its time. As might be expected, his grasp of speech mechanics was also advanced. He divided the sounds of speech into four classes—vowels, sibilants, semivocals, and consonants—and with approximate accuracy described the articulation of each. The vowels, or "clear contoured sounds" as he called them, were produced, for example, "by the streams of air passing from the lungs in respiration through the larynx; which is furnished with many small muscles, which by their action give a proper tension to the extremity of this tube." He compared the opening and closing of the glottis to the trumpet stop of an organ, and experimented with reproducing such sounds by blowing through the windpipe of a goose.

One of his most ingenious inventions was a "speaking machine," for which he developed a phonetic alphabet. It had a wooden mouth with lips of soft leather, a valve for nostrils that could be manipulated by hand, and a larynx consisting of a length of silk ribbon stretched between two slats of wood. A bellows supplied the air, which caused the ribbon to vibrate "much like a human voice" between the wooden sides. Although the machine was never completed, it convincingly simulated several speech sounds, and when the leather lips were gradually closed, even produced "a most plaintive tone." A bit grandiloquently, Darwin imagined that it might some day be built in gigantic form, large and loud enough "to command an army or instruct a crowd."

At home, Darwin communicated with his household staff through a sort of intercom or speaking tube that connected his study with the kitchen. One day, we are told, "a local yokel who had brought a message, being left alone, was terrified to hear a sepulchral and authoritative voice from nowhere demand, 'I want some coals.' "Thinking such a request (disembodied yet distinctly at his ear) could only come from the devil, he dropped the message he had brought at once and ran.

Not incidentally, Darwin's grandson Charles thought that stuttering was inherited. He thought so because he stuttered slightly himself, his grandfather had stuttered, and so had his uncle, for whom he was named. This other Charles (Erasmus's eldest son) was sent by his father to France with a tutor when he was a child, in the hope that if he didn't speak English for a time the impediment might disappear. Upon his return, he continued to stammer in English but was fluent in French. Information about the stutter of the more famous Charles is scarce. One anecdote has it that because of his speech he did so poorly in school that his father told him severely, "You will be a disgrace to yourself and all your family." Later on it reportedly discouraged him (ironically enough, in light of his challenge to Creationism) from considering a career in the Church.

# Chapter Five

The nineteenth century gave rise to a prodigious literature on stuttering, and new theories abounded. Some of these were advanced; others were merely newfangled, and resurrected (or degraded) older versions of themselves.

The French were perhaps the most industrious. In 1817, Jean Marc Gaspard Itard, a French physician associated with the Institute for the Deaf and Dumb in Paris, suggested that stammering was "caused by a general debility of the nerves which stimulate the movements of the larynx and tongue." To repair the tongue's muscular weakness, he recommended gymnastic exercises for it, and also invented a little fork made of gold or ivory to support the tongue during speech. This was to be worn inside the alveolar arch of the lower jaw. By his own admission, it led at first to "confused and indistinct" articulation, yet he could not say how long it should be worn. His patients, it seems, never had a chance to stutter, because whenever the device was removed (as at night or at mealtimes) they were forbidden to speak at all.

In 1829, another physician, Serre d'Alais, diagnosed the disorder as a "nervous affection" that resembled, on the one hand, "chorea of the muscles which modify the sounds," and on the other "a tetanic rigidity of the muscles of phonation and respiration." He was thus the first to clearly distinguish between repetition and blocking. But his prescription was crude: brisk pronunciation, to be accompanied by a vigorous shaking of the arms. "You must shake the stutterer by the arms at every syllable," he advised parents and other therapists, "or he may do it himself, and he will be surprised at the facility which these motions give him." Both speaking and shaking were to be done in rhythmic time to a metronome-like instrument of his own devising called an isochrome.

In the same year, a colleague, Antoine Rullier, advanced the theory that "the cerebral irradiation which follows thought, and puts the vocal and articulating organs in action, gushes forth so impetuously and rapidly, that it outruns the degree of mobility possessed by the muscles concerned, which are . . . left behind." The result is the "convulsive and spasmodic state which characterizes stuttering." This idea (really a version of the perennial notion that stutterers think faster than they can speak) was also more appealing than his cure, which was to cauterize the integument covering the hyoid bone.

In 1830, the surgeon Hervez de Chegoin reverted to the more simplistic theory that "the cause of stuttering consists either in the shortness of the tongue or the vicious disposition of the frenum, which fixes it to the inferior part of the mouth, and thus restricts its motions." His solution, of course, was to divide it, but (perhaps inspired by Itard's fork) in some cases he also proceeded to "double the dental arches by inserting a silver arch behind the lower incisors," to bring them nearer the tongue.

In 1831, Columbat de l'Isère, a prominent authority, followed d'Alais in distinguishing between repetition and blocking, and recommended breathing exercises and rhythmic speaking, to be paced by his own "muthonome."

In England, therapies emerged with the same haphazard mix. Dr. Joseph Frank in his *Practice of Medicine,* published in 1810, assumed stuttering to be a depraved habit and thought regular beatings might help. Other documented (if otherwise incredible) remedies included ingesting a Finnish insect repellent normally rubbed on cows, bleeding the lips with leeches, and eating the feces of goats! Certain medieval medical procedures (now divorced, however, from the humoral doctrine that had made them intelligible) also remained, such as blistering the tongue.

In 1835, Dr. H. M'Cormac announced his "discovery hitherto made by none. The patient endeavors to speak when the lungs are empty, and cannot." His simple remedy (today called "airflow") was to breathe deeply and speak as the breath was exhaled. Similarly, Sir Charles Bell in his *Philosophical Transactions* (1832) identified the problem as one of intonation and concluded that the stutterer was trying to speak on insufficient air. His prescription was phonetic drill. A decade later, Marshall Hall, in *Diseases of the Nervous System,* blamed stuttering on an emotional disposition, and prescribed cathartics and "speaking in a subdued, continuous tone, first dilating the thorax."

Hall's emphasis on thoracic breathing was of course all

wrong; by contrast, G. Niel Arnott, in the *Elements of Physics, and Natural Philosophy* (1864), showed an understanding of laryngeal blocking that was approximately correct. Since, as he thought, the vocal cords were paralyzed by extreme contraction, the aim should be to keep them vibrating—for example, by droning any simple sound. Beyond that, he recommended that words "be joined together, as if each phrase formed but one long word, nearly as they are joined in singing; if this be done, the voice never stops, the glottis never closes, and there is, of course, no stutter."

Benjamin Beasley (who seems to have run a quite popular clinic in pastoral surroundings outside London) likewise emphasized that by locking the glottis, compressing the lips, or jamming the tongue against the teeth or gums, the stammerer was "trying to speak in an impossible manner." "How utterly foreign to free speech is all effort," he noted; since the mechanism had "to run smoothly and softly, like a well-oiled machine."

Another substantial theory was developed by the phrenologist Andrew Combe, and set forth in his favorable review of the *Causes and Cures of Stammering* by Felix Voisin, which appeared in the Edinburgh *Phrenological Journal* in 1826. To begin with, he briskly disposed of the notion that the vocal apparatus of the stutterer, including his tongue, was in any way malformed. Quoting Voisin, he noted that the tongue was "not larger than [that of] other people, nor its ligaments laxer, nor its frenum excessively long, nor the teeth so placed as to present any obstacle," and that whenever such abnormalities occurred they did not cause stammering but permanently affected pronunciation. Stammerers, on the other hand, could be perfectly fluent—when enraged, for example, they might swear profusely without impediment. "But passion," he wrote, "can never remove a physical cause, make a large tongue small, set crooked teeth straight, or tighten the ligaments of the tongue." The real cause, he concluded, lay in irregular signals transmitted from the brain that disrupted the normal muscular coordination of speech.

To substantiate this, he drew an analogy between the chronic condition of stuttering and stuttering due to stage fright, which he ascribed to "a *conflict* between the *desire* to speak well, and the fear of speaking ill"—a theory close to that of Erasmus Darwin. His general conclusion was: "Wherever two or more diverging purposes of nearly equal power assail the mind, and prompt to opposite courses of action at the same time, there stammering appears." He found the therapeutic example of Demosthenes compelling, for with a mouth full of pebbles, he had to concentrate on the very particular movement of his articulators to speak "without choking himself or allowing the pebbles to drop from his mouth." A complete cure was possible only when, by dint of diligent practice, the muscles involved became accustomed to working in the proper way.

Although Combe saw a resemblance between chronic and accidental stuttering, his observation that stutterers sometimes demonstrate perfect fluency in moments of excitement helped distinguish the disorder from its colloquial prototype. One of his contemporaries, James Hunt, likewise scoffed at the idea that anger (or any other strong emotion) necessarily exacerbated the problem, and told the following amusing anecdote to illustrate his point:

In January, 1833, three gentlemen, Monsieurs Dub . . . , Mart . . . , and Ou . . . , stutterers to a painful degree, went to the French Academy of Sciences, for the purpose of being examined before a commission prior to the commencement of their treatment. . . . On leaving the Academy, they entered a tobacconist shop to purchase some cigars. Mr. Dub . . . , who was the least timid, commenced his address, "Dooo do doo donney mois des ci des ci des cigarres." It so happened that the tobacconist was himself a terrible stutterer; he was thus by no means surprised to have found a comrade in affliction, but he was certainly far from imagining that the other two were similarly affected. When, therefore, the tobacconist asked, "De-dede-de-dedequel quel qua-qua-qu qua qualité vou-vou-voulez vous les-les cigarres," and the others then began to stutter horribly as well, the tobacconist, thinking himself mocked, flew into a violent rage, seized a stick to beat them, and swore at them in the most energetic terms, without the least impediment in his speech.

In the United States, perhaps the most capable discussion of stuttering could be found in an article by Edward Warren, the Harvard surgeon, published in the *American Journal of Medical Science* in 1837. Like Combe and Voisin, Warren realized that there was no inherent defect in the speech apparatus itself, and regarded stuttering as a neurological disorder aggravated by circumstance. "Stammering," he wrote, "originates in a weakness of the nervous system—an irregular action of the nerves. Afterwards, the fear of stammering causes a person to stammer; the organs of speech soon acquire a depraved habit; the nerves also are habituated to irregular action, as in chorea, and the habit may become difficult to eradicate, even if the mental cause is removed." He then proceeded to give the first thoroughgoing account of the phenomenon of word substitution:

I may allude to another thing also which gives a singular appearance to the conversation of the stammerer, even when he appears to speak with ease. . . . Without being perfectly aware of it himself, he is constantly considering before he speaks whether the words he means to employ are easy to articulate. . . . Hence, he makes use of odd and outre expressions; and as no two words are perfectly synonymous, the words he substitutes for those which would more perfectly express his meaning, and which are chosen in haste, and for no other reason than easy utterance, often sound odd or convey a meaning very different from what he wishes. Although he may see that this is the case, yet exhausted by the effort he has already made, he does not attempt to correct the impression he has communicated. In this way he may very readily obtain the character of an idiot or an imbecile.

Warren's understanding of fluency in singing was equally acute. Noting that "the sound is continued from syllable to syllable, and word to word," without interruption, he recognized the promise of therapeutic methods that "prolong the sound in this manner. . . . So long as the stammerer can [do this], he can speak with ease; his great difficulty is in the commencement of a sentence and in avoiding interruption in breaking the sound into syllables."

Warren, Combe, Voisin, and a handful of others stood head and shoulders above their colleagues. Overall, speech therapy in England and America fell into the hands of elocutionists, who relied on respiratory, vocal, and articulatory drills.

Rather typical of this approach was that of Andrew Comstock, a professor at the Vocal and Polyglott Gymnasium in Philadelphia, who in *A System of Elocution, with Special Reference to Gesture, to the Treatment of Stammering and Defective Articulation* (1841), prescribed rhythmic speaking, and the recitation of material designed "to be spoken with explosive force; for example, 'Satan's speech to his legions,' " from Milton's *Paradise Lost*. Beyond that, he commended vigorous exercise to work off tension, saltwater bathing, antispasmodics, and body rubs. So long as the patient had a cheerful yet determined disposition, and a good ear, he thought the prognosis was good; but if he was melancholy and irresolute, or unable to carry a tune, not much could be done for him.

Within a short time, throughout the United States there was a proliferation of privately owned speech schools that charged large fees for guaranteed cures. Most of the cures involved gimmicks—such as feet stamping, finger snapping, drawling, or the use of a singsong voice. One required patients to place their tongue in some peculiar position, another to keep the jaw clenched during speech. Alexander Melville Bell, whose son invented the telephone, held that stuttering was the result of misaligned teeth, and prescribed speaking "while biting down firmly on the blade of a paper cutter." More highly publicized was a method devised by a New York physician named Yates, and afterward adopted and promoted by a Mrs. Leigh. This required the patient, while speaking, to keep the tip of his tongue in contact with his palate on the upper alveoli just behind his upper teeth. How this could produce any kind of intelligible utterance is hard to imagine, but it was to be done even at night, when a small roll of linen was placed under the tongue. Packaged as a secret cure, Leigh's "American method," as it was called, was introduced into Germany and Holland by an aptly named Monsieur Malebouche, who sold it in turn to the governments of Belgium and Prussia.

However unhelpful, such gimmicks appear innocuous beside the brief but horrible reversion at this time to tongue surgery. Since the days of Aristotle (as we have seen) the tongue had been regarded as the chief organ of speech; and (at least since Galen) the frenum the part controlling its mobility. During the eighteenth century, interest had begun to shift from the frenum to the tongue's underlying nervous organization, together with the idea that "vibrations" (or nervous impulses) flowed through the nerves. It was suspected that stuttering might be a nervous disorder in the sense that such impulses were not being adequately transmitted to the speech muscles from the brain. This seemed to explain why stutterers had particular trouble in initiating sounds, "because there the Organs pass in an instant from Inactivity to Action, whereas the subsequent parts of words and sentences may follow the foregoing from Association." Under the influence of such notions (in themselves advanced), radical surgery as a cure for stammering was introduced in 1841 by a Prussian surgeon and professor of clinical surgery at the University of Berlin, Johann Friedrich Dieffenbach. Hypothesizing that stammering was caused by a spasm of the glottis that communicated itself to the tongue as a lingual cramp, his operation consisted of making a horizontal section at the root of the tongue, and excising a triangular wedge across it so that the impulses could get through. This was far more drastic than dividing the frenum; yet it failed to give pause.

Meanwhile, a new and careless distinction had arisen between "stammering" and "stuttering" as clinical terms. In the past, the two had been used interchangeably, and at least through the Renaissance had tended to appear together (in the rhetorical habit of doubling) as synonyms. "Her felow did stammer and stut," wrote the poet John Skelton in 1529; and in 1688, Randle Holme in *The Academie of Armoury* defined the disorder this way: "A Man . . . [doth] Stammer, Stut, when the Voice or Words come not freely, that hath an

Impediment in his Speech." In the eighteenth century their alternate use occurred without distinction, but by the early 1800s, under the influence of the new educational emphasis on "right speaking," some had begun to define stammering as "a defective articulation of certain sounds"—a very different problem with which stuttering became confused.

Not knowing any better themselves, several hundred stutterers (including some mere "stammerers") submitted themselves to the new operation. All in some way were maimed or mutilated; and several actually died.

Dieffenbach, however, was not a charlatan. He had already made a name for himself with successful cleft-palate surgery (which helped pave the way for modern achievements in plastic surgery), and had subsequently treated strabismus, or spasmodic squinting, by severing tendons connected to the muscles of the eye. He had first performed that operation in Berlin in 1839, and its success led him to consider the therapeutic possibilities of an analogous operation on the tongue. "The idea lately suggested itself to me," he explained, "that an incision carried completely through the root of the tongue might be useful in stuttering which had resisted other means of cure, by producing an alteration in the condition of nervous influence, allaying the spasms of the chordae vocales. . . . The obvious way of doing this was to make a transverse section of the tongue."

On January 7, 1841, Dieffenbach decided to put his hypothesis to the test. His patient was a thirteen-year-old boy whom he sympathetically described as

highly intelligent and talented, but who had stuttered from his earliest childhood, and to so painful an extent, that the defect was thought to be quite incurable. It varied, however, much in degree; when at the worst, he was unable even to produce a sound. He stuttered in Latin and French, as well as in his own language—sometimes on one set of words, and sometimes on others. . . . The presence of a stranger invariably affected him in a manner most painful to behold. His face became distorted; the alae of the nose worked convulsively; his lips moved quiveringly up and down; his eyelids were expanded into a wild and eager stare; the tongue was now stiff, now played convulsively within the mouth; and the muscles of the throat, larynx, and trachea were sympathetically affected. Thus, after terrible efforts, the boy gave utterance to a mangled and imperfect word.

He next graphically described the procedure:

The patient was seated in a high chair opposite the window; his head being held perpendicular by one assistant, who at the same time drew the angle of his mouth backwards by means of retractors. His tongue being thrust forward was seized by a pair of strong forceps (furnished with teeth to prevent their slipping) which I gave to another assistant to hold. By these means the tongue was steadied and compressed transversely. Having seized the tongue posteriorly to the forceps, with the thumb and forefinger of my left hand I compressed it transversely and at the same time elevated it; then passing a long, curved, pointed scalpel from the left side beneath the tongue and at the posterior half, until I felt the point at the right side with my forefinger, I cut directly upwards, dividing the tongue right through. I now grasped the tongue in front of the wound with a pair of strong forceps, armed at the point with teeth, pressed it firmly together, and with a small, straight scalpel, made a section from above downwards . . . by these two sections a piece the shape of a wedge was cut out of the tongue at its posterior half. The wound was now united by six ligatures of thick silk, which were passed in such a manner as to encircle in depth and breadth a considerable portion beyond the margin of the wound, and were forcibly drawn together in order to restrain the hemorrhage. The patient became rather faint toward the termination of the operation, and afterwards vomited large quantities of blood he had swallowed. As soon as we had washed his mouth out with water, I was exceedingly pleased to hear him pronounce words which, previous to the operation, he was unable to articulate.

The first thing he said distinctly was "There is some blood running down my shirt."

This operation was performed without general anesthesia, two years before ether was introduced. In subsequent procedures, Dieffenbach varied his technique, and when not excising a wedge, opted for a transverse myotomy in the root. But so convinced was he of its pioneering importance, that he at once dashed off an account of it to the Institut de France. His exhilaration was tempered only by the obvious trauma the patient had endured, and he recommended it not be performed on anyone unless their cardiovascular and nervous systems were strong enough to bear the shock and loss of blood.

Even before an official announcement was made to the French medical establishment, word leaked out and the operation was celebrated in the popular press. Surgeons were "immediately beset with sufferers desiring treatment," and they "responded to this demand." In France, several of the more reputable rushed to claim some precedent for themselves. On February 6 in Paris, just one month after Dieffenbach's own first operation, Charles Phillips, a Belgian, performed two. By the end of April, two other French physicians, Alfred Velpeau and Jean Amussat, had operated on a hundred patients between them, willfully introducing their own variations—Velpeau snipping off parts of the tongue, without always excising a sublingual wedge; Amussat cutting here and there at surrounding tissue and muscle, including that of the lower jaw. To stem the bleeding, which was generally profuse, they tried packing the mouth with ice, or applied sponges soaked in vinegar. If that didn't work, they cauterized the wound.

Not to be outdone, still another colleague, Baudens, came up with his own operative technique. This involved nothing more than stretching the frenum with a hook, then plunging the points of a sharp pair of scissors into the muscles on either side, and snapping them shut.

The surgical craze spread to England, where Bennett Lucas, a London physician, began to divide and partly remove muscles which opposed "the free elevation of the tip of the tongue to the superior alveolar arches." A colleague, James Yearsley, imagined that stutterers were short of breath because their swollen tonsils and uvula blocked their throat. And so he decided to cut them out. So eager was he to be heralded as the true innovator that he wrote to a leading medical journal to say he had been "taken by surprise when the Memoir of Professor Dieffenbach appeared. I had been aware of my principal facts for two months previously and was silently endeavoring to bring the subject to maturity. Professor Dieffenbach states that he performed his first operation upon the tongue January 7th, 1841; while I had performed mine upon the throat as early as December 5th, 1840." Over the course of the next couple of months, Yearsley operated on about forty stammerers, all of whom, he subsequently announced, appeared wild with joy at their instantaneous cure. However, another doctor who independently interviewed several of them commented wryly that they merely "stammered out that they were better."

Meanwhile, there had been little peer review, and almost no attempt to verify the surgeons' claims. Then on May 17 one of Amussat's patients died; soon thereafter, another victim succumbed in Berlin. Reports of a recrudescence of stuttering in dozens of patients began to appear. By then the highly respected English medical journal *Lancet* had gone on the attack:

> Within the last few months, a perfect mania for operating seems to have seized the profession . . . not content with bringing some hundreds of squinting eyes straight (a few being put out or destroyed in the attempt), we now have operators who straighten the crooked back by cutting out a portion of its motor muscles, who remove false anchylosis of the knee by dividing the hamstring tendons, and who set a crooked head straight by cutting across the sterno-cleido-mastoideus. . . . The last grand series of the bold and violent operations serve as the climax. Dieffenbach, Amussat, and others have brought forth operations for the cure of stammering, as if the nervous impediment of speech depended on a mechanical obstruction. . . . The frightful attendant hemorrhage, the great risk of losing the tongue, or life itself, has little to recommend it.

Nevertheless, many reputations were at stake and the practice was not completely repudiated until year's end. By that time, however, it had been taken up by country doctors (not always of the wise and folksy kind), in whose hands it would survive.

No known cures were obtained. In some cases, there may

have been temporary relief, either by autosuggestion, a by-product of muscular exhaustion, or simply because the patients were distracted by their pain. Perhaps all had to speak rather slowly and deliberately at first, for obvious reasons, which usually helps. Among the maimed, moreover, were several who had a strictly elocutionary problem and hadn't really stuttered at all.

Surgery, of course, can be mere butchery, or art. In this instance, its primitively simplistic cure for stuttering, like the contemporary experiments in curing clubfoot by dividing the Achilles tendon, or treating other deformities from wryneck to crooked fingers by tenotomy, form part of the notorious and sorry background to Flaubert's famous parody of all such operations in *Madame Bovary.*

As for Dieffenbach, he took the long view. Optimistic that the procedure, if nothing else, would contribute to the development of surgical instruments, he predicted: "We shall have conical and oblique incisions, from the surface and under the skin! We shall have knives and scissors with improved curves, and a thousand variously fashioned forceps and hooks." Notwithstanding his otherwise respectable place in medical history, his name, in uncomplimentary fashion, has been given to the common houseplant dieffenbachia, or dumbcane—so called because its stalk contains oxalates that can render a person speechless from inflammation of the tongue and throat.

Over the years, other surgical remedies have been tried, including removal of the adenoids, widening of the dental arch (which came into vogue in the early 1920s), and even, occasionally, trepanning, or cutting a hole in the skull. In 1898, for example, it is reported that a Romanian surgeon by the name of Ionnesco trepanned a fourteen-year-old stutterer "who had a very asymmetrical skull, the left half of it being rather flat. Ionnesco cut out a large bone-flap on the left side and incised the dura mater. Immediately the cortex herniated through the incisions and a large quantity of cerebrospinal fluid flew out." Aphasia followed, and three days later blood clots had to be removed. According to Ionnesco, the aphasia then cleared and the boy was cured—although no confirmation could be had of that fact.

During this whole period, lots of bizarre gadgets and devices were patented for therapeutic use. Most of these were horrific-looking appliances furnished with springs and wires and screws. Some were designed to prevent the teeth from being clenched; others, in the event of clenching, to keep the breathing passages open by means of a tube. Still others (veritable face masks) gripped the articulators so that they couldn't move at all. One inventor came up with a slotted V-shaped metal clamp for the tongue, which weighed it down in such a way as to compel the wearer to speak slowly. Another, with an orthodontic-like device furnished with a sharp projection for pricking wayward motions of the tongue. Even more annoying was a contraption to be worn around the chest and equipped with a plunger attached to a spring. When a full breath had been taken, the plunger was released and began to prod the wearer to begin to speak.

Ingenuity knew no bounds. During the glossotomy craze, *Lancet* reported a cure that combined radical surgery with a kind of bioelectrical hookup. The patient's coccyx was removed and a needle with a large eye inserted "into the cancellated structure of the bone." Whenever the patient wished to speak, he attached the wire of a small galvanic battery to the needle, and the current, conveyed up the spine, kept the soft palate "distended like a sail, and the uvula floating like a pennant upon its stream."

How pretty to picture; how appalling to conceive.

One of those who adamantly opposed the new tongue surgery (and the gadgetry then coming into vogue) was James Hunt, a distinguished ethnologist with extensive medical training, who in 1861 published a landmark examination of the affliction based in part on the work of his father, Thomas, a well-regarded therapist. Hunt accepted the new distinction between stammering and stuttering, but he did not confuse them; and in general represented the state of contemporary understanding at its best.

Stammering, he wrote, was poor enunciation; stuttering, characterized by frequent repetitions of initial or other elementary sounds, and always more or less attended with muscular contortions. He realized that the entire speech apparatus—respiratory, vocal, and articulatory—had to work in tandem; and understood perfectly the operation of the larynx in the production of voice.

Noting that stutterers can usually sing, whisper, and speak fluently when alone, he ascribed the first to rhythmic breathing, the second to not having to coordinate the laryngeal muscles with articulation, and the third, to the ease of solitude.

Finally, he noted the possible inheritability of the disorder, given that many sufferers "have a parental or collateral relation labouring under the same infirmity . . . [and] many instances can be adduced where the defect has descended for several generations." His own therapy, however, was based on the idea that speech is largely unconscious and that once the automatic habit of it had been lost it could never be regained. Accordingly, he endeavored to teach his patients "to speak consciously, as other men speak unconsciously," not only by physical practice but by cultivating "mental tranquillity and self-control."

One of the stutterers Hunt worked with was Lewis Carroll; but it is curious how little of contemporary theory and practice is actually reflected in the struggles of most of the celebrated men and women—Charles Lamb, Leigh Hunt, Charles Kingsley, Clara Barton, and Henry James, among others—of whom we have some account.

Whether or not Charles Darwin's impediment dissuaded him from considering a career in the Church, it is certain that the English essayist and critic Charles Lamb was thus prevented from proceeding with his education, first to the university level and then to the priesthood, as he'd hoped. Instead, he was obliged to leave school at the age of fourteen and eventually found employment as a clerk in the East India Company, where he remained for much of his life.

On the face of it, this was a disaster for him. Lamb hated the everyday routine, felt he had been "defrauded" of any chance to pursue his scholastic inclinations, and found himself belittled at work for his cultural interests and tastes. Yet the everyday routine was probably therapeutic for him. He was prone to depression and neurasthenic ills, and at age twenty-one briefly committed himself to an insane asylum. From the age of twenty-two, his life was substantially taken up with the care of his sister, Mary (ten years his senior), who had murdered their mother with a bread knife. Under such circumstances, having to get up in the morning and do something practical (however much he may have resented it) was probably a blessing in disguise. At the same time, for a modicum of work, as Thomas De Quincey observed—chiefly auditing the account books for wages and pensions—he was well maintained for thirty-three years by his clerkship, ultimately enjoyed a retirement arrangement that he himself termed "magnificent," and was able to pursue an active literary career. Indeed, a fair amount of his writing, it seems, was done on company time.

Lamb's regular promotions at work also increased his self-confidence, as he himself remarked. Meanwhile, he wrote *A Tale of Rosamund Gray* (a prose romance), *John Woodvil* (a poetic tragedy), *Tales from Shakespear* (a retelling of the plays for children), a similar rendition of Homer's *Odyssey*, volumes of *Essays of Elia* (his pseudonym), and hundreds of letters of a literary kind.

Lamb's disposition was evidently so amiable that even the schoolmates of his youth had indulged his infirmity of speech. As an adult he often "grunted once or twice" before beginning to speak, and then his words came out "in little explosive bursts." Nothing, however, could curb the volubility of his wit. Once, when sitting near the door of a London bus, a would-be passenger stuck his head in and asked, "All full up inside?" "Oh yes," exclaimed Lamb, "th-th-that last p-p-p-piece of p-ie, qu-qu-qu-qu-qu-qu-quite f-finished me!"

Lamb drank quite a bit (chiefly gin), and smoked heavily, which he found to be "a solvent of speech." As the clouds of smoke billowed upward, "the ligaments which tongue-tied him," he wrote of himself, "were loosened, and the stammerer proceeded a statist!"

. . .

Lamb's friend and colleague, Leigh Hunt, whose parallel career as an essayist, critic, and poet has often led them to be paired, attended the same school (Christ's Hospital) and was unable to advance for the same reason. As he explains, "I hesitated in my speech. . . . It was understood that a Grecian [the rank of an advanced student destined for the university] was bound to deliver a public speech before he left school, and to go into the Church afterwards; and as I could do neither of these things, a Grecian I could not be." At the age of fifteen, with "a vague sense of worldly trouble, and of a great and serious change in my condition," he left school to try to make his way in the world. He found employment as a clerk in the War Office, but after a few years used his savings to start the weekly *Examiner* with his brother John. A mouthpiece for liberal reform, it vigorously attacked the government in a series of articles that culminated in a rash editorial that ridiculed the Prince Regent (afterward King George IV) as a "fat Adonis of fifty." For that gross indiscretion, Hunt was prosecuted for libel, fined, and imprisoned for two years.

His sentence brought to an abrupt end an idyllic and somewhat idle style of life. By his own account, "I did nothing for the greater part of the week but write verses and read books. I then made a rush at my editorial duties; took a world of superfluous pains in the writing; sat up late at night, and was a very trying person to compositors and newsmen." The conditions of his incarceration, however, were not severe. His family was allowed to live together with him in quarters he was free to furnish as he pleased, and which he transformed into a quaint sort of bower. The walls were papered over brightly with trellises of roses and the ceiling painted blue with white clouds like the sky. He had all the books he could read, a pianoforte, and surrounded himself with the plaster busts that had adorned his study at home. In prison, he and his wife also conceived their third child. To some degree his plight even helped make his career. He was quickly adopted as a martyr for the liberal cause, and Lamb, Hazlitt, Byron, Shelley, Jeremy Bentham, and others all came to pay their respects.

For all that, his confinement took its toll. Hunt's nature was timid, his health naturally delicate (as a child he had suffered from "almost every disorder to which infancy is exposed"), and after his release, we are told, "his morbid fear of cowardice and his habit of seclusion were so strong upon him that for months at a time he would not venture out into the streets." He also assumed a less polemical stance on matters of public debate, and devoted more time to writing verse. Poverty and debt shadowed him in his later years, during which he was ironically sustained by royal grants and government pensions, as well as an annuity from Shelley's son.

Those inclined to believe that a dominant and overprotective parent tends to foster a shy, physically awkward, and stuttering child may claim their paradigm in Hunt. Although his father was an irrepressibly cheerful alcoholic for whom debtors prison was almost a second home, his mother gave him, in his own words, such "an ultra-tender and anxious rearing," as to make him fearful of life itself. Like Lamb, he was plagued early on by nightmares, "sighed compulsively," and was followed by anxiety and depression throughout his life. Unlike Lamb, however, Hunt's impediment was not indulged at school. "The worse my stammering, the worse the ill-treatment," he bitterly remembered, and he especially dwelled on the day when the master of the school, infuriated by his repetitions, struck him on the mouth with the *Iliad* and knocked out a tooth.

Although Lamb and Hunt were prevented from becoming clergymen by their speech, Charles Canon Kingsley, the English orator, writer, and chaplain to the queen, was not. After graduating from Magdalene College, Cambridge, he was ordained as curate of Eversley, and two years later became the parish priest. A "Christian Socialist" preoccupied with the evils of industrialism, he eventually rose to become chaplain to Queen Victoria, canon of Westminster, and professor of modern history at Cambridge. He also wrote didactic social novels, historical novels with an anti-Catholic bias, and *The Water-Babies,* a popular children's book inspired by Darwin's theories of evolution and natural selection.

Kingsley attributed his stammer to, alternatively, his overbite and "nerves ruined by croup and brain fever in childhood." He recommended dumbbell exercises to strengthen the lungs, a "manly" diet of beef and beer, and sports like boxing to build up fortitude. He also thought it helped to place a bit of cork behind the back teeth. In school, his nickname (according to a great aunt) was "the Cave, on account of his large mouth, which seemed all the larger as it gaped in search of an elusive word." Although he enjoyed a privileged education, he came to resent the fact that his upbringing was as sheltered as it was, believing that the rough and tumble of a public school might have cured him of his affliction. Nevertheless, he boasted that it never affected him in the pulpit or at his prayers, and (rather vainly) claimed it humbled his vanity, and kept him from being glib at soirees. "I could be as great a talker as any man in England, but for my stammering. I know it well," he tells us. "When a man's first thought is not whether a thing is right or wrong, but what will Lady A or Mr. B say about it, depend upon it, he wants a thorn in the flesh."

If "speaking for God" (to use Kingsley's own presumptuous phrase) were explanation enough as to why his impediment temporarily disappeared, Moses ought not to have had any difficulty, and Lewis Carroll, I suspect, wouldn't have had as much trouble as he did.

The third of eleven children, Carroll was born Charles Lutwidge Dodgson on January 27, 1832. In addition to his stutter (an impediment shared by two other siblings), he was deaf in one ear as a result of childhood mumps. When he was thirteen, he wrote a charming parody of Victorian didactic verse in which his speech defect was given pride of place:

> Learn well your grammer,
> And never stammer,
> Write well and neatly,
> And sing most sweetly,
> Drink tea, not coffee;
> Never eat toffy.
> Eat bread with butter.
> Once more, don't stutter . . .

Carroll's father was a curate, and (fulfilling his own inclination as well as his father's hopes), after completing his schooling he was ordained a deacon in the Church of England. He intended to become a priest, but ultimately judged himself unfit for parish work. Nevertheless, he often involved himself in clerical duties and the Church remained central to his life. At Christ's Church, Oxford, he enjoyed a successful academic career as a tutor in mathematics and developed into an accomplished photographer; but it was his literary work, undertaken at first as an avocation, that immortalized him as the endlessly inventive and witty author of *Alice's Adventures in Wonderland, Through the Looking-Glass, The Hunting of the Snark* (a narrative nonsense poem), *Sylvie and Bruno,* and other works. As their author, he adopted the pseudonym of Lewis Carroll, from a Latinization of his first and middle names.

Carroll's upper lip often trembled when he spoke, but by cultivating a slow and deliberate style of speech, he was eventually able to preach with some confidence before a congregation. His sermons were always composed in advance with great care, but never written out, as he preferred to preach from notes. "By this means," writes a biographer, "he preserved the illusion of perfect extempore delivery" even though he had gone over the material repeatedly until he knew it by heart. His presentation was highly organized, as one parishioner vividly recalled: "Looking straight in front of him he saw, as it were, his argument mapped out in the form of a diagram, and he set to work to prove it point by point, under its separate heads, and then summed up the whole." Carroll was adept at word substitution, and extemporizing allowed him latitude; but the impression of poise he gave was dearly won. "A sermon would be quite formidable enough for me," he once admitted, "even if I did not suffer from the physical disability of hesitation; but with that super-added, the prospect is sometimes almost too much for my nerves." Sometimes it was. On October 31, 1862, he recorded a humiliating instance in his diary: "Read service in the afternoon. I got through it all with great success, till I came to read out the first verse of the hymn before the sermon, where the two words 'strife, strengthened' coming together were too much for me, and I had to leave the verse unfinished." Five years later he was struggling with no more success: "Read the first verse in the afternoon with a good deal of hesitation. I must try what more practice can do." A decade or so before he had consulted with James Hunt, whose therapeutic advice had been helpful; but it did not suffice. In 1872, he therefore sought the help of a certain Dr. Lewin in Nottingham, and with rekindled hope sat through a three-hour lecture-explanation of his cure.

Whatever it was, it failed.

Carroll's stutter, however, seldom troubled him when talking to children, and he acquired many child friends. His Alice tales were inspired by Alice Liddell, daughter of the dean of Christ's Church, who with her two sisters occasionally went on picnics, boating excursions, and other outings with him. Always chaperoned, as he insisted, they also visited him in his college rooms. Many years later, Alice charmingly evoked the scene:

We used to sit on the big sofa on each side of him, while he told us stories, illustrating them by pencil or ink drawings as he went along. . . . He seemed to have an endless store of these fantastical tales, which he made up as he told them, drawing busily on a large sheet of paper all the time. They were not always entirely new. Sometimes they were new versions of old stories; sometimes they started on the old basis, but grew into new tales owing to the frequent interruptions which opened up fresh and undreamed-of possibilities.

Other child-friends were similarly enchanted, including the sons of the poet Alfred Lord Tennyson (one of whom stammered), and the children of George Macdonald, another writer of children's tales.

Carroll, of course, was aware of the appearances, and when one of his sisters wrote to him about it with some concern, he replied:

> I think all you say about my girl-guests is most kind and sisterly. . . . But I don't think it is at all advisable to enter into any controversy about it. . . . My experience is that the opinion of "people" in general is absolutely worthless as a test of right and wrong. The only two tests I now apply to such a question as having some particular girl-friend as a guest are, first, my own conscience, to settle whether I feel it to be entirely innocent and right, in the sight of God; secondly, the parents of my friend, to settle whether I have their *full* approval of what I do.

The most egregious case of psychologizing in the literature on Carroll may be found in a book by Richard Wallace, in which literally every single phrase in Carroll's work is perversely interpreted as an anagram confessing a psychosexual and/or masturbatory fantasy. Wallace assures us that Carroll's life was "a nightmare of constant inner turmoil on the verge of psychic destruction," and that he was "incapable of loving" and devoured by "all-consuming hate." Through cryptic clues, his Wonderland reveals "the destructive world of coercive parenting, the violent world of the English public school system, the worlds of pornography and erotica, homosexuality, sexual perversion, of stuttering, migraines, and insomnia." His explanation for the freedom with which Carroll could speak to children is, of course, sinister: he had them under his control.

Other biographers also analyzed his stutter without illumination. One thought it had something to do with his rejection of Holy Orders (even though he had begun to stutter as a child!); another, that it was a deliberate device to set himself apart from the adult world. James Joyce presciently warned in *Finnegans Wake* against overconstruing Carroll in this way: "And so wider but we grisly old Sykos [psychos, i.e., psychoanalysts] who have done our unsmiling bit on 'alices, when they were yung [Jung] and easily freudened."

Like Joyce, Carroll delighted in all sorts of word games. He liked to form a sort of verbal looking glass by reversing the letters of a word ("evil is the opposite of live"), and playfully indulged in like-sounding combinations of syllables with a different sense—as when the Mad Gardener in *Sylvie and Bruno* says "wriggle early" for "regularly." More famous are the "portmanteau" words Humpty Dumpty defined: " 'Slithy' means 'lithe' and 'slimy.' 'Lithe' is the same as 'active.' You see it's like a portmanteau—there are two meanings packed up into one word." Other delightful examples are "gallumphing" (galloping in triumph) and "chortle" (chuckle and snort). In the evolution of the language, a number of common words, of course, have been born of such blends: for example, "twirl" (twist and whirl), "smog" (smoke and fog), and "brunch."

Stutterers, it may be noted, occasionally blend words by accident, and Carroll's happy invention may have begun with a verbal mishap. On the other hand, his improvisations may just as easily owe something to his tendency (as a mathematician) to "toy with statistical permutations," as one scholar points out. Nevertheless, stuttering itself, by discreetly painful allusion, did find its way into his work. In *Alice,* for example, he introduced himself as Dodo—a stammering repetition of the initial sound of Dodgson, his surname; and in his story *A Tangled Tale,* a schoolteacher is unkindly nicknamed by his pupils "Balbus," Latin for stammerer.

Another writer whose style was almost unquestionably affected by his impediment was Henry James.

Born on April 15, 1843, in New York City, James spent a somewhat itinerant childhood in the care of tutors and governesses (in both Europe and the United States), grew up shy and bookish, and at the age of nineteen enrolled in Harvard Law School. He had a pronounced stutter, which he had inherited from his father, and in a letter to Ralph Waldo Emerson (dated November 17, 1843), Thomas Carlyle had this to say of the elder Henry James: "He confirms an observation of mine, which indeed I find is hundreds of years old, that a stammering man is never a worthless one. Physiology can tell you why. It is an excess of delicacy, excess of sensibility to the presence of his fellow-creature, that makes him stammer."

Whether sensibility had anything to do with the younger Henry's stutter or not, it didn't provide much consolation. In law school, to his humiliation and dismay, his infirmity prevented him from assuming the role of a courtroom advocate in a classroom demonstration of a trial; and on one occasion he simply "collapsed into silence"—an incident he felt shame about for years. By 1870, he had begun publishing stories in magazines, wrote his first novel in 1875, gave up the law, and moved to Paris where he made the acquaintance of Turgenev, Zola, and Maupassant. Subsequently, he settled in London, where he became a fixture of society, a much-invited guest to "the great Victorian houses and country seats," and was elected to London clubs. Yet "his manner," in the words of Edmund Gosse, was always "a little formal and frightened, which seemed strange in a man living in constant communication with the world." His stutter had a good deal to do with that, as may be surmised from the impressions of a number of people belonging to the circle in which he moved. "Henry James," recalled one emphatically, "could not say a sentence without repeating himself"; others made note of his "hesitant 'm-m's,'" "ers," "ahs," and so on, and the regular drumbeat of his hand on the table, which evidently helped him to get the words out. Ruth Draper, an American actress, found unforgettable "the anguished facial contortions" that accompanied his speech, and the socialite Elizabeth Jordan tells us that James "almost invariably broke up his sentences into little groups of two, three, or four words, and repeated each group three times." She recounted the following episode as typical in this respect:

> The scene was the London dinner table of Colonel and Mrs. George Harvey at Claridge's Hotel. Mr. James and I had met that evening for the first time and he had taken me into dinner. . . . One of our fellow guests was Henry Savage Landor, the explorer. Mr. Landor's experiences in Tibet, during which he was supposed to have been tortured by the natives whose forbidden city of Lhasa he had penetrated, were not many years behind him . . . [but] I had met several leading Londoners who expressed to me the greatest doubts of the accuracy of Mr. Landor's memories . . . and I ventured to ask of Mr. James, who had evidently met him several times, whether he shared these doubts.

"Eliminating – ah – (very slow) eliminating – ah –eliminating nine-tenths – (faster) nine-tenths of-of-of (very fast) what he claims (slower) of what he claims –of what he claims (very slow) there is still – there is still – there is still (very much faster) enough – left – e-nough left (slower) to make – to – make – to – make – a remarkable record (slow) a remark – able record, (slower) a remarkable record (very slow).

James could be witty in conversation, but (due to his hesitations) was not good at repartee. His whole conversational manner, in fact, according to the writer Desmond McCarthy, "was largely composed of reassuring and soothing gestures intended to allay, or anticipate, signs of impatience" with his speech.

Elizabeth Jordan, not incidentally, used to imitate James's stutter as a parlor piece ("the most popular of my social monologues," she gaily conceded); but what might be comprehensible (if not excusable) in a society matron, is rather disappointing in Virginia Woolf. In a letter to Violet Dickenson on August 25, 1907, she mockingly wrote:

We went and had tea with Henry James today, and Mr and Mrs [George] Prothero, at the golf club; and Henry James fixed me with his staring blank eye—it is like a child's marble—and said "My dear Virginia, they tell me - they tell me - they tell me - that you - as indeed being your father's daughter nay your grandfather's grandchild - the descendant I may say of a century - of a century - of quill pens and ink - ink - ink pots, yes, yes, yes, they tell me - ahm m m that you, that you, that you *write* in short." This went on in the public street, while we all waited, as farmers wait for the hen to lay an egg.

Others, however, found their patience well rewarded, and assumed they had been privileged to witness a great writer's agonized but uncompromising search for the *mot juste*. As one admirer put it: "In conversation he was meticulously careful to convey his precise meaning, so that his remarks became a sort of Chinese nest of parentheses; it took him some time to arrive at his point but he always reached it, and it was always worth waiting for." As a result, rather generous and respectful allowances were made for the repetitions and hesitations that delayed his journey along the way:

> The greatest compliment that can be paid to that subtle, complex mind of his is that, notwithstanding his mannerisms and hesitations that would be so tediously unbearable in the case of most of us, Henry James never came even near to being a bore. One had to wait a long time for the thought to be expressed; one watched the process of its germination and development; but when it came one felt that it had been tremendously worth waiting for, and that it was a thought peculiarly his own and expressed as no other man could have expressed it.

Of course, James did not always stutter, and his acquaintance Gertrude Atherton remembered occasions when "he talked as if every sentence had been carefully rehearsed; every semi-colon, every comma, was in exactly the right place, and his rounded periods dropped to the floor and bounced about like tiny rubber balls."

The truth is that James's hesitations and circumlocutions sometimes reflected his search for the *mot juste,* and sometimes nothing but his painful struggle to speak. The only one who seems to have understood what was really going on was his intimate friend, and perhaps artistic equal, Edith Wharton:

His slow way of speech, sometimes mistaken for affectation—or, more quaintly, for an artless form of Anglomania!—was really the partial victory over a stammer which in his boyhood had been thought incurable. The elaborate politeness and the involved phraseology that made off-hand intercourse with him so difficult to casual acquaintances probably sprang from the same defect. To have too much time in which to weigh each word before uttering it could not but lead, in the case of the alertest and most sensitive of minds, to self-consciousness and self-criticism; and this fact explains the hesitating manner that often passed for a mannerism. . . .

Wharton then movingly recounted an evening when his mask fell away:

I had never heard Henry James read aloud—or known that he enjoyed doing so—till one night some one alluded to Emily Brontë's poems, and I said I had never read "Remembrance." Immediately he took the volume from my hand, and, his eyes filling, and some far-away emotion deepening his rich and flexible voice, he began:

Cold in the earth, and the deep snow piled above thee,
Far, far removed, cold in the dreary grave,
Have I forgot, my only Love, to love thee,
Severed at last by Time's all-severing ways?

I had never before heard poetry read as he read it; and I never have since. He chanted it, and he was not afraid to chant it, as many good readers are, who, though they instinctively feel that the genius of the English poetical idiom requires it to be spoken *as poetry*, are yet afraid of yielding to their instinct because the present-day fashion is to chatter high verse as though it were colloquial prose. James, on the contrary, far from shirking the rhythmic emphasis, gave it full expression. His stammer ceased as by magic as soon as he began to read, and his ear, so sensitive to the convolutions of an intricate prose style, never allowed him to falter over the most complex prosody, but swept him forward on great rollers of sound till the full weight of his voice fell on the last cadence.

James's reading was a thing apart, an emanation of his inmost self, unaffected by fashion or elocutionary artifice. He read from his soul, and no one who never heard him read poetry knows what that soul was.

That chanting style also gave a rhythmic boost to his speech (like the drumbeat of his hand in conversation) while in dictation, he found the rhythmic clatter of an old Remington typewriter an indispensable aid. One of his secretaries, in fact, noticed that he was unable to dictate to the sound of quieter models, but, "exactly like" a singer at the piano, had to be accompanied by a rhythmic response.

James's last great novels were composed (or written) by dictation, and Leon Edel, author of the standard James biography, has speculated that their increasingly allusive style might have something to do with that fact. The resemblance between dictation and James's conversational style, with "its amplifications, hesitations, and interpolated afterthoughts," was also noted by Desmond McCarthy and others at the time, including the writer E. F. Benson, who perhaps expressed it best:

Nothing would be further from the truth than to say that he talked like a book, but most emphatically he talked like a book of his own in the making, just as he used to dictate it, with endless erasures of speech, till he got the exact and final form of his sentences. Just so in his talk he tried word after word to express the precise shade he required. . . .

Not only did James make a virtue of necessity, he found virtue in it, for (remembering Edith Wharton's speculation) he turned his hesitations and prolongations into opportunities for deeper thought.

From such literary complexities, the life of Clara Barton, founder of the American Red Cross, offers some surcease. Barton suffered from a stutter or lisp that was relatively mild and that she eventually controlled by holding her mouth in a somewhat rigid position—"stabilizing her articulators," as a contemporary therapist might say. But in her childhood it caused her much embarrassment, and in her autobiography she recalls the laughter of other children when she mispronounced words.

Born Clarissa Harlow, she was timid as a child and traced her fearfulness to a number of traumatic childhood events. Like Lamb, she suffered from nightmares and (also like Lamb) the shadow of mental illness hung over her after her sister, who was given to violent rages, attacked their brother with an axe.

When she was fifteen, the direction of her life was unexpectedly determined by the pronouncements of a phrenologist. After carefully surveying the moral and intellectual geography of her head, he declared: "She will never assert herself for herself; she will suffer wrong first. But for others she will be perfectly fearless. Throw responsibility upon her." This was interpreted by her family as meaning that she should teach. She did that for many years, before embarking on the humanitarian work that would earn her fame. She organized a relief agency for the wounded during the Civil War, tended casualties under fire at Second Bull Run, the siege of Charleston, Fredericksburg, and other battles, and at the special request of President Lincoln set up a bureau of records to help locate the missing-in-action. As a result of her efforts, she became known, affectionately, as the "angel of the battlefield." In 1869–70, while vacationing in Europe, she was drawn into relief efforts for the Franco-German War, and after working for the International Red Cross, founded, in 1881, its American branch.

# Chapter Six

The future of stuttering therapy would ultimately derive from a more complete understanding of neurophysiology and the brain. But the road to its epiphanies would prove a winding one, and as the twentieth century dawned, confusion reigned. To begin with, the nomenclature itself had become even more chaotic. Some defined stuttering as a physical, stammering as a psychological problem; others, stammering as an inability to voice, and stuttering as a spasmodic repetition of sounds. Still others considered stuttering a hesitation on consonants, and stammering a hesitation on vowels. The elocutionists and the parlayers of gimmick cures held sway. The substantial insights of Darwin, Combe, Voisin, Warren, Hunt, and a few others were almost completely lost sight of; and into the intellectual vacuum stepped psychoanalysis.

Stuttering is troubling—anyone who stutters is bound to be troubled by it; so it was inevitable that a condition exhibiting so many symptoms resembling neurotic behavior would attract theorists of mental disease.

Well before Freud, of course, there were those who regarded stuttering as a personality disturbance or "nervous disorder" of some sort, and from the mid-nineteenth century on, while the French, English, and Americans were preoccupied for the most part with physical concepts, the Germans had adopted a more psychological approach. Generally speaking, they regarded it as an anxiety neurosis—a "phonophobia" or fear of speech (as one therapist put it in 1830); and this pre-Freudian view of the problem would, in fact, prove more pertinent than what psychoanalysis expounded in its wake. Among the leading German theorists, Karl Ludwig Merkel, a professor of medicine at Leipzig University, described stuttering in 1842 as a "failure of confidence in the ability to communicate"; this notion was adopted and expanded by Reinhold Denhardt, who wrote in 1890: "If we examine the mental processes during stuttering, we see that the disturbance typifies the struggle between two opposing forces. The volition which tries to convert the thought into speech is pitted against the belief that we are unable to accomplish what we intend. One drives, the other restrains." Merkel and Denhardt acquired adherents, and some American physicians took up the theme. One, E. W. Scripture, described stuttering in 1912 as a learned response become habitual and maintained by anxiety.

Other psychological theories had a different bent, and perhaps the most curious and original was advanced by C. S. Bluemel. In *Stammering and Cognate Defects of Speech* (1930), he hypothesized that stammering was a form of transient auditory amnesia—that for some reason the stutterer is unable to recall the sound image of the vowel he wishes to enunciate. Almost as peculiar was an idea of Emil Froeschels, a distinguished Viennese physician, who at about the same time suggested that since chewing motions were the basis of the muscular action used in articulated speech, the stutterer should practice "chewing his own breath" as he spoke.

Freud himself, not incidentally, was unwilling to treat stutterers since (in his view) psychoanalysis had failed to cast light on the disorder. But a number of his disciples were less circumspect. Some hypothesized infantile repressions of an erotic nature, or fixations at the oral or anal stage of childhood development; others a conflict between the superego and the id; or an ambivalence about speaking due to "unspeakable" feelings or thoughts. One such theorist was Knight Dunlap, who put the matter this way: "The boy who has no great fear or scruple about letting out his gutter vocabulary . . . never . . . becomes a stammerer, but the boy who is carefully brought up . . . a stammerer of the deadlock type. He is always fearful of letting out some obscenity! . . . It is the proper little boys who become stammerers." Still others, of course, believed that stuttering expressed the memory, wholly or partially repressed, of some painful event.

Fixation theories predominated, however; and taking their cue from a passing speculation made by Freud in a letter to Ferenczi in 1915 that stuttering might have something to do with a conflict over excremental functions, a number of analysts supposed that it converted "the vocal and buccal opening into a sphincter." Since normal speech implied "the act of giving out, of expulsing something of oneself into the outside world," stuttering, and especially blocking, must by analogy represent constipation in some form.

More influential was a theory advanced by Isador H. Coriat, a Boston physician who concluded that stuttering was a severe psychoneurosis caused by the "persistence into adult life of infantile nursing activities." His remarkable elaboration of this idea bears detailed review as an example of a theory that can begin (at least on its own terms) with a plausible premise, and then progressively detach itself from the reality of the object of its thought.

Dismissing all other theories out of hand, he begins:

> In the pregenital stage [of libido development] there are two important phases that enter into the stammering neurosis, namely, the earlier oral stage and the later anal-sadistic stage. This earlier stage, with its sucking and biting movements, can be demonstrated in practically every stammerer. If the motor accomplishments of the attempts to speak are carefully observed, the stammerer will be seen in the act of nursing at an illusory nipple, as shown by the sucking movements of the lips and tongue, the excessive flow of saliva, deep breathing, rapid heart beat, and yawning, all followed by a feeling of relaxation after the enunciation of the difficult word.

Supplementary possibilities occur to him: "Stammerers will often bite the tongue and the mucous membranes of the mouth to the extent of bleeding when they attempt to speak, a symptomatic cannibalistic feature that is a remnant of the early and primitive oral sadism." This enables him to confidently announce that a stutterer's anxiety has nothing to do with speaking per se, but is "a protective mechanism to prevent complete betrayal of the primitive oral and sadistic tendencies through speech."

Every aspect of the condition is then forced within this frame. When, in a paroxysm of stuttering, the speaker grinds his teeth and experiences uncontrollable spasms of the jaw, he is, according to Coriat, actually reexperiencing "primal sexual pleasure," for "he chews the words and luxuriates in their sounds and this prolonged oral possession tends to annihilate the word through compulsive repetition in the sucking and biting of syllables." Increased salivation while struggling to articulate reproduces that of the nursing infant, and his "peculiar hand movements" become the very gestures made by an infant "when it wants to be fed" or "cleaned after excreting."

From this sucking-sadistic paradigm, Coriat also derives both the character of the alphabet and explanations for the relation of the stutterer to each sound. The labial consonants ("p," "b," and "m") he says are repeated more often than others because the muscles used to produce them are the same exercised in nursing at the mother's breast. And the repetitions sometimes seem to go on forever because "no matter how frequently a stammerer repeats, a complete sensation of oral gratification is never produced because the (unconscious) wish to gratify the oral libido is so strong, that it is not absolutely satisfied in the repetition."

Since the stutterer, by definition, is stuck in a nursing state, it almost goes without saying that he has an Oedipal complex, and (because of his mother fixation) is "a latent homosexual."

Stuttering in women is related to the castration complex: "The tongue has become a displaced phallus," and the stuttering expresses both "the wish to have a phallus, and the wish to incorporate it by a cannibalistic tendency. . . . In the deep analysis of female stutterers, there emerges, under considerable resistance, a combination of phallic disgust and phallic envy. Chronologically, the original castrator is the mother, and as a consequence female stammerers, as part of the Oedipus situation, hate their mothers."

Perhaps "under considerable resistance" is the operative phrase.

Even more strangely, Coriat concludes that stutterers by nature are "optimistic"—"their whole attitude towards life shows that they expect the mother's breast to flow for them eternally." That's why stammerers "are always hopeful of attaining normal speech and go from cure to cure." He even finds them gregarious, "for the reason that their narcissistic and egoistic tendencies are gratified in social activities." Since melancholy and shyness are so often apparent in stutterers (as universally remarked since ancient times), and Coriat can find only proof of pleasure in their pain, one might be excused for wondering if he ever met a stutterer in his life. But of course he met, and treated, many, and many others were treated applying his ideas.

Indeed, such theories had become commonplace in psychiatric circles by 1928. Over the years they would prove quite useless in analysis, and one might have expected them to fade from the scene. But like the hypothetical infant they imagined, they clung to their first sustenance; and dogmatic variations of them can still be found today in psychiatric handbooks in common use.

While psychoanalysis was groping for relevance in this area, a revolution in stuttering therapy was taking place at universities of the American Midwest.

At the University of Iowa, Samuel Orton (a more grounded psychiatrist) advanced the intriguing hypothesis that stutterers were naturally left-handed or ambidextrous, and had been forced to change their handedness in childhood in order to conform to the social norm. Since (as it was known) the brain's left hemisphere controls the muscles on the right side of the body, and the right hemisphere those on the left, to force a left-handed child to be right-handed could conceivably cause hemispherical confusion—with stuttered speech as the result. This idea was taken up and developed by Orton's colleague, speech pathologist Lee Edward Travis, who concluded that stuttering was due to the lack of any clear dominance over speech functions by one of the two hemispheres. Either the dominance was incomplete, or there was a conflict of dominance between the two; in either case, the theoretical result was that the usually synchronized arrival of nerve impulses to the paired speech musculatures of centrally located structures (like the tongue, lips, and jaw) was incorrectly timed. This supposed, as one authority put it, that "the dominant hemisphere determined the precise moment when both hemispheres would fire their impulses to the right and left sides of the speech mechanism."

A participant in one of the experiments conducted in the 1930s to test the hypothesis recalled:

Needle electrodes were inserted into the paired jaw muscles of a stutterer, one on each side of his face. While he talked freely or stuttered, the little electrical currents accompanying the nervous impulses to these muscles were amplified and photographed. As one of the guinea pigs, I recall not only the needles but also the atmosphere of delighted discovery that filled the laboratory when it was found that during my occasional spells of normal speech the nervous impulses arrived regularly in both the right and left jaw muscles, whereas they came down to only one of those muscles when I stuttered. Other stutterers showed the same results. Normal speakers had perfectly synchronized nervous impulses even when they pretended to stutter very badly.

Nevertheless, the results, proved inconclusive over time, and other ways of confirming the hypothesis were tried. These included (in the recollection of another participant) "simultaneous talking and writing; vertical board writing; rhythm practice with jaw bite, tongue protrusion, and panting; abandonment of two-handed activities such as typing and piano-playing, and use of the preferred hand wherever possible" in order to reestablish the margin of dominance on the right side of the brain. Indeed, with the very righting of their brains at stake, some stutterers went so far as to have their right arms placed in casts, or bound up in slings or leather restraints.

At about the same time, at the University of Wisconsin, Robert West was formulating his equally novel theory that the disorder was akin to epilepsy, and manifested itself in tiny stress-related "pynknoleptic" seizures that disrupted speech. The stutterer was said to be peculiarly vulnerable to these convulsions because he possessed an underlying neuromuscular condition called dysphemia—"an inherited predisposition for the breakdown of the central mechanism that controlled speech functions." Others (for example, E. J. Boome and M. A. Richardson, in their book on *The Nature and Treatment of Stuttering*) similarly opted for the view that certain children "inherit peculiar neuropathic tendencies which predispose [them] to stammering."

Meanwhile, the character of the stammer itself was getting some imaginative attention. If it could not be overcome (and few seemed able to overcome it), perhaps there were ways in which it could be modified.

The first to advocate voluntary stuttering of any sort was Bryng Bryngelson, a professor at the University of Iowa, who based his approach on the idea that the best way to overcome a vicious habit was to practice it deliberately. Assuming that stuttering was learned behavior, he thought that by stuttering in a highly conscious and controlled fashion, with slow repetitions, the sufferer would no longer be dealing with an uncontrollable event.

Bryngelson's two most famous disciples were Charles Van Riper and Wendell Johnson, whose approaches, as they matured, would dominate speech pathology for the next fifty years. The two men had quite a lot in common: both had been born and raised in the rural Midwest; both stuttered severely to the point of being incapacitated; and both had been exploited by the gimmick cures of "stammering schools." In fact, they had both attended (though not at the same time) the Michigan stammering school of Benjamin Bogue, who had taught them to speak in a drawling chant while rhythmically swinging dumbbells. Later, they ended up together at the University of Iowa, where they began to find their way.

Johnson had originally come to Iowa City to meet Lee Edward Travis, to whom he quickly revealed the dimensions of his plight:

A few days after I arrived, Dr. Travis asked me to come with him to one of his classes. He explained that he wanted the students to observe my speech. I sat in a chair beside his desk at the front of the room. There were thirty or forty students looking at me. Dr. Travis told them who I was and that I was from a small town in Kansas and then he handed me a book and asked me to read aloud to the students. I read for five minutes—and got out four words.

With utter dedication, Johnson set out to reestablish what he presumed to be his lost left-handedness and the hemispheric dominance to which it belonged. But "ten years and countless bruises later," he wrote, "having become a threat to my own thumbs, I placed in storage my many ingenious braces and mittens . . . put away my left-handed scissors, and with my right hand wrote 'Finis' to the experiment, still stuttering splendidly."

With similar commitment, Van Riper had had electrodes planted into the muscles of his face, tied up his right arm in a sling, wrote vertically, panted, and so on, but was just as unsuccessful in this phase of his quest.

Meanwhile, both had also been following Bryngelson's counsel to stutter deliberately, and over time each came up with new modification techniques—Van Riper with the "slide," and Johnson with the "bounce." The slide involved prolonging the initial sound of a syllable; the bounce, its voluntary repetition, in a relaxed and easy way.

Not long ago, at the age of eighty-five, Van Riper recalled the circumstances under which his idea was born:

[It] came to me while hitch-hiking my way home from Rhinelander, Wisconsin, where I had spent a month as the hired man on a farm, pretending to be a deaf mute because my stuttering was so severe and grotesque I could not get any other employment. I had hoped thereby to be able to live without talking, but after a month I couldn't bear it any longer and left to return to a home where I felt I would not be welcome.

After walking several miles I sat under a tree to rest near a field where a man was plowing. Soon an old man in a Model-T Ford pulled up beside me and he got out to talk with the farmer. I noticed that he had an odd way of speaking with many little hesitations but I didn't think it was stuttering. When they finished their conversation, I accosted him with the thumb gesture for hitch-hiking and he told me to get in the car. Then of course came the inevitable question: "What's your name, son, and where are you going?" Oh, how I stuttered when I tried to tell him with gasping, facial contortions and body jerks!

The old man then explained to him that he had been a stutterer all his life, and over time had learned to stop fighting it, and instead just "let the words leak out." Van Riper divined from this that his own task was to find a way of stuttering "that would be tolerable both to others and myself . . . to stutter so easily and effortlessly that it wouldn't matter . . . to change it to a more fluent form."

In addition to the slide, Van Riper developed other techniques for coping more effectively with blocks. Through thoughtful self-observation, he noticed that, whereas the articulators of a normal speaker are in constant motion, stutterers tend to prepare for a feared sound by tensing them in place. Moreover, when a stutterer repeats a particular sound, he is actually not having trouble with it—after all, he's repeating it!—but with moving on to the rest of the word. Accordingly, he advised him to relax the articulators and keep them mobile; refrain from struggling should a block occur;

and (if it did) try to glide out of it with a prolongation of the sound. Once out, he should repeat the word as a "post-block correction" in a more relaxed way.

While Van Riper elaborated his slide, Johnson developed his bounce, which eventually assumed three forms: the "whispered bounce" (or quiet repetition of a word until it could be spoken without tension); the "phrasal bounce" (or repetition of the initial sound of each phrase); and the "thought bounce" (or repetition of a sound in thought before speech).

In short, the former emphasized ways of making speech smoother and more continuous, the latter relied on varieties of controlled repetition to make the stutter itself less pronounced. Beyond that, both urged their patients to confront their fears and no longer avoid situations where they expected to block. Van Riper also stressed that the impediment could not always be measured by its overt physical manifestations, and identified the "interiorized stutterer" as one who, though often fluent, was constantly on guard against any revelation of his disability. Johnson, for his part, sought to change the stutterer's attitude. "Stuttering is not something that happens to you," he told his somewhat baffled clients. "It is something that you do."

Johnson remained at Iowa; Van Riper, in the late 1930s, left to found a speech clinic and research center at what is now Western Michigan University.

Van Riper's approach remained more or less consistent over the years; Johnson, deeply disillusioned by the failure of the cerebral dominance and dysphemia theories to prove that stuttering had an organic cause, restlessly sought other explanations, and his thinking continued to evolve. In the following decade, he startled the profession with his wholly different diagnosogenic theory, which faulted the home environment, as epitomized by his famous pronouncement that "stuttering begins not in the child's mouth, but in the parent's ear." In holding parents responsible, Johnson took his inspiration from the speculations of two contemporary psychiatrists, Froeschels and Bluemel, who thought that the early (but not necessarily normal) hesitancies and repetitions in a child's developing speech could be neurologically fixed in place by a parent's overanxious and stern correction. Bluemel, moreover, optimistically suggested that if the child were left alone, he would probably grow out of it; but if he were unhelpfully reproved, he would become self-conscious, fearful in his anticipation of faltering, and by struggling not to stutter, find himself ever more entangled in its coils.

Johnson, a bit more dogmatically, suggested that stuttering actually began with attempts by parents to correct *normal* disfluencies, which they inappropriately labeled "stuttering." The disorder, in other words, was caused by its diagnosis. In this scenario, the child, in order to meet his parents' unrealistic speech expectations, tries not to make mistakes, and by trying not to, does. The harder he tries, the more he fails, and the more self-conscious he becomes. Even though there is nothing inherently wrong with his speech, he now becomes aware of himself as a stutterer, and secondary struggle characteristics arise.

It had long been obvious (even to elocutionists) that circumstance could aggravate the disorder—for example, Oskar Guttmann (an elocutionist) had warned in 1893 that "nothing is more adapted to promote stuttering than terror and fear." Johnson's theory also resembled another hypothesis that a person could "catch" the disorder by making a conscious effort not to. Boome and Richardson (in their book alluded to above) had argued that any critical response by others in response to a purely accidental block, "by drawing attention to the mechanism of articulation, induces further consciousness of what should be an automatic action." In order to avoid repeating his mistake, the child tries not to block again "and further impediment results."

Based on Johnson's theory, the incidence of stuttering might be expected to increase in proportion to the competitiveness of the environment in which children were raised. So his adherents looked around for confirmation of the fact. It was supposed, for instance, that many more men than women stuttered because there was more pressure in Western societies for males to succeed. Some psychiatrists had already considered stuttering in this light, as an illustration of civilization and its discontents. One in 1923 had quaintly discriminated between the sexes in this way:

> The female has more control of her speech but a smaller vocabulary. The male tends to be more quiet and silent but more aggressive in his thoughts. The female talks about simpler things, encounters less criticism. Present-day competitive civilization leaves little time for speech to the male, while at the same time he must use all his mental efforts. The female, on the other hand, has no need for involved thinking, as she is in constant close relationship with the simple human being, the child. She can cook, bake, crochet, and talk at the same time.

Predictably, the search also began for civilization's opposite—the idealized, nonstuttering aborigine. "All travelers," James Hunt had written in 1861, "who have long resided among uncultivated nations, and whose authority is of any weight, maintain that they never met with any savages labouring under an impediment of speech." Though skeptical himself, Hunt thought (if true) it must be due to "their freedom from mental anxieties and nervous debility, the usual concomitants of refinement and civilization." Lo and behold, soon after Johnson's diagnosogenic theory was formulated, reports came back from anthropologists in the field that no instance of stuttering, or word for it, could be found among the Bannock and Shoshone Indians of southeastern Idaho, where indulgent parenting was beyond anything later espoused by Dr. Spock. When stuttering was subsequently documented among the far more competitive Indian tribes of the northwest Pacific Coast, it seemed only to prove the point.

Other anthropologists became curious, and fanned out. The Bannock and Shoshone peoples were more thoroughly interviewed, and it so transpired that they were quite familiar with stuttering and had a number of words for it besides. Then evidence turned up of a high incidence of stuttering among children of the Accra district of the Gold Coast, and among the Bantu it was found that the sex ratio of male to female stutterers was about four to one: the same as for societies in the West. Words for stuttering that had existed before the advent of whites were also identified by philologists in all the major African language groups.

Johnson's theory may have helped promote a more tolerant home environment; but its chief legacy (aside from the guilt it imposed on countless parents) was that stuttering was basically psychological in origin, or "learned avoidance behavior." This was taken up by the speech pathologist Joseph G. Sheehan, and elaborated into an approach-avoidance complex beyond what Erasmus Darwin or Combe had conceived. Like Van Riper and Johnson, Sheehan stuttered badly, and had become a therapist as the result of his own quest for a cure. Although he shared his colleagues' emphasis on the modification of stuttered speech, he concentrated more on the condition's psychodynamics. In his view, the stutterer constantly oscillates between the desire to speak and the desire to avoid speaking, and, depending upon the relative strengths of these two drives, stutters to a lesser or greater degree. He subsequently transformed this into an interpretation of stuttering as a self-role conflict. "Stuttering," he wrote, "is a disorder of the social presentation of the self. Basically, stuttering is not a speech disorder, but a conflict revolving around self and role, an identity problem." He pointed out that sufferers are sometimes fluent in non-self roles—when adopting foreign accents, say, or acting in a play—but tend to have particular trouble with self-referent words such as "I" or "my," or with their own names. In Sheehan's view, the stutterer, once past childhood, could find no way out of his dilemma than "to become a stutterer all the way, through self-acceptance in this role." Accordingly, he forcefully attacked any therapeutic approach that aimed at fluent speech: "The experience of speaking normally may set up a role expectation for fluency, and actually lead to more stuttering. On the other hand, when the individual stutters and thereby enacts more fully the role of stutterer, the fear-producing role expectations for normal speech are diminished. In this manner enactment of the stutterer role leads to fluency, and vice-versa."

By putting so much stress on eradicating the psychology of avoidance, Sheehan came up with some startling ideas. One was that blocking actually reduces fear, because once it happens, there is less anxiety about hiding the fact that it might. And he argued that the slide, for example (developed to overcome blocks) should be chiefly used on *nonfeared* words, so that it didn't become a crutch.

Sheehan's observations about words of self-reference found broader reflection in the theory that stuttering generally occurs on words with significant content—that stuttering occurs on words, not sounds. The writer Elizabeth Bowen, for example, consistently blocked on the word "mother," after her mother's death. On the other hand, she stuttered on many other words besides, and W. Somerset Maugham (as a contrary literary example) was just as likely to stutter on prepositions and conjunctions as nouns and verbs. In fact, it has been found that lists of neutral words— numbers, for instance—can evoke as much stuttering as a weighted text.

John Updike's ideas on the psychology of the disorder, not incidentally, bear some resemblance to those of the Sheehan school. "It happens when I feel myself in a false position," he tells us (Sheehan often called it a "false role" disorder); or (as Updike put it in a recent interview): "You stutter, I think, when you can't feel the ground under your feet." In his memoir he offers two examples: when as class president of his high school he had trouble making a speech because "I did not, at heart, feel I deserved to be class president . . . and in protest at my false position my vocal apparatus betrayed me"; and when at a meeting of the American Academy and Institute of Arts and Letters "I tried to read through a number of award citations . . . I had not written. I could scarcely push and batter my way through the politic words." His self-exploration, however, turns up other factors that precipitate it too: fear of certain audiences—for example, those he expects to be critical; guilt, or being "in the wrong," as with the "sharp and painful stutter" he developed with his own children after his marriage broke up; and in talking with such strangers as "a bored and hurried electrician" over the telephone. (Updike's electrician is like Larkin's postal clerk.)

About the time that Sheehan's theories were taking shape, behavioral psychology came into vogue, and operant conditioning (which postulates that behavior can be modified by its consequence) was applied to the malady. Loud blasts of tone were administered to the ears of subjects every time they blocked, or painful shocks by means of electrodes strapped to their legs or wrists. The results of such experiments proved inconclusive; meanwhile, the anxiety neurosis theory had undergone a revival, to be redescribed now as an "anticipatory struggle reaction." Advanced with eloquence and precision by Oliver Bloodstein, Professor of Speech Pathology at Brooklyn College, it basically holds that stutterers stutter because they think some special effort in speaking is required. Therefore "if a stutterer were to forget that he was a stutterer, he would have no further difficulty with his speech." Bloodstein illustrated the idea by a simple analogy: "Almost anyone would be able to walk the length of a wooden plank without stepping off if the plank was on the ground. But put the plank fifty feet in the air, and it becomes an entirely different matter. . . . If someone were to inquire of us why we weren't walking normally, we would have to say it was because we were trying to keep from falling off."

An interesting psychological picture of the stutterer may also be found in the work of Dominick Barbara, who allows himself to get caught up in a tenuous theory about a "Demosthenes complex," but then fortunately returns to more demonstrable psychological truths. "Confused and embarrassed by his apparent failure to control his speech apparatus," he writes, "the child eventually accepts the notion that there is something deeply wrong with him." Alienation becomes the core of his personality, and an inner futility grows into an absence of hope. "He may feel that the world should provide him special services and privileges and entitle him to a position in life, a job suitable to his speech incapacity, and make allowances for his stuttering." In this way, his neurotic needs become claims, even as he is driven into imposing impossible "shoulds" upon himself.

Although Barbara attempts to construct a psychological type, it has never been possible, in fact, despite a good deal of psychological testing, to establish that a stuttering personality exists. In 1939, for example, a researcher at Columbia University incorporated into his thesis on *The Personality Structure of Stuttering* a comically inclusive list of "neurotic tendencies" or "personality peculiarities" stutterers were said to display:

| | |
|---|---|
| Shyness | Pampering |
| Egocentricity | Moodiness |
| Introversion | Rebelliousness |
| Hysteria | Masochism |
| Anxiety | Irritability |
| Finickiness | Moroseness |
| Insomnia | Taciturnity |
| Fear | Neurosis |
| Dextrosinistrality | Restlessness |
| Infantilism | Jealousy |
| Negativism | Exhibitionism |
| Hypochondria | Compensation |
| Submissiveness | Undemonstrativeness |
| Obsession | Worry |
| Nagging | Unreasonableness |

More disciplined surveys have shown that at least before secondary struggle behavior sets in, stutterers are psychologically no different from anyone else. They are not inherently neurotic or disturbed, and every sociodisjunctive attribute associated with the disorder (such as lack of self-confidence, social reticence, feelings of hopelessness, and so on) can best be explained by the stuttering itself, as its consequence. Indeed, "it is remarkable," observes John Paul Brady, Professor of Psychiatry at the University of Pennsylvania, "how well adjusted most severe stutterers are, given the nearly constant anguish and stress many experience in their daily efforts to communicate."

Concepts of adjustment are relative, of course, and one wouldn't want to generalize along these lines too far. The "claustrophobia, isolating fear, and searing episodes of humiliation," as Edward Hoagland puts it, that stuttering brings in its wake, are bound to leave their mark; and most, if not all, of the notable men and women described were certainly troubled in their own way. On the other hand, even Arnold Bennett, the prolific English novelist, playwright, critic, and essayist who enjoyed tremendous popularity in the early decades of this century, managed despite a stutter that was extraordinarily severe.

Born into modest circumstances in the pottery district of Staffordshire, Bennett did moderately well in school but after failing his law examinations twice, took up writing. He worked for a time for a woman's magazine, and in 1898 published his first novel, *A Man from the North*, when he was thirty-one. "I began to write novels because my friends said I could," he once stated. "The same for plays. But I always had a feeling for journalism." Over the next quarter-century or so he wrote numerous novels, stories, essays, travelogues, and other occasional pieces, before dying of typhoid fever in March of 1931.

Bennett rarely revealed anything of his personal life even in his letters, but his mother thought his stutter could be dated from the time he fell out of his high chair and struck his head on the floor. H. G. Wells speculated about a psychosexual problem of indeterminate origin: "I think there was some obscure hitch in his make-up, some early scar that robbed him of the easy self-forgetfulness, that 'egoism expanded out of sight,' of a real lover. I associate that hitch with the stammer that ran through his life. Very far back in his early years something may have happened, something that has escaped any record, which robbed him of normal confidence and set up a life-long awkwardness." Even so, Bennett married twice, and with his second wife he had a child. Whereupon he sold his yacht ("You can't have a baby and a yacht," he wrote) and seems to have enjoyed a fairly stable family life.

His stutter, however, remained beyond control. According to his friend W. Somerset Maugham, "it was painful to watch the struggle he had sometimes to get the words out. It was torture to him. Few realized the exhaustion it caused him to speak. What to most men was as easy as breathing, to him was a constant strain. It tore his nerves to pieces. Few knew the humiliation it exposed him to, the ridicule it excited in many, the impatience it aroused." Bennett sought help from a variety of speech therapists, as well as a hypnotist, but without relief. Not long before his death, Maugham encountered him at a London party, sitting on the floor and "beating his knee with his clenched fist to force the words from his writhing lips."

Margaret Drabble, the English novelist and one of Bennett's biographers, suggested that "the hesitancy of his speech made him more direct and incisive in his prose." Maugham's nephew similarly claimed that his uncle's stutter "made his prose pithy, crisp, and succinct." No doubt an incentive to be brief helps develop a talent for brevity, although Henry James stands as an incontrovertible argument against all such platitudes. In any case, Maugham, unlike Bennett, had a good deal to say about his own impediment, and its impact on his life. In *Ten Novels and Their Authors* he tells us: "I have no doubt that a physical or spiritual disability affects the character of an author's work. To some extent it sets him apart from his fellows, makes him self-conscious, prejudices him, so that he sees the world, life and his fellow-creatures from a standpoint, often unduly jejune. . . ." And in *A Writer's Notebook,* he applied this to himself:

> I think many people shrink from the notion that the accidents of the body can have an effect on the constitution of the soul. There is nothing of which for my own part I am more assured. My soul would have been quite different if I had not stammered or if I had been four or five inches taller. I am slightly prognathous; in my childhood they did not know that this could be remedied by a gold band worn while the jaw is still malleable; if they had, my countenance would have borne a different cast, the reaction towards me of my fellows would have been different too.

Maugham's earliest years were spent in Paris, where his mother was married to an English solicitor attached to the British embassy. She died when he was eight, and his father when he was ten, whereupon he went to live in Whitstable, Kent, with his uncle, the local vicar. In the following year (1885), he was enrolled in King's School, Canterbury. When he was taken to meet the headmaster, he asked his uncle to tell him about his stammer in advance. Perhaps he hoped the whole school would also be informed. If so, it didn't do him much good. He was often teased, and he especially remembered an occasion when he was asked to stand and construe a passage from the Latin, and his stuttering provoked uproarious laughter in the room. His teacher, having to shout to make himself heard, banged on the desk and said: "Sit down, you fool! I don't know why they put you in this form!"

On another occasion he went up to London with his uncle, who decided to stay the night but sent Maugham home. Maugham went off to the station with money for his ticket, and got in line. When he came to the window, he couldn't pronounce "Whitstable," and after a long time trying the people behind him began to get impatient and "suddenly," he recalled, "two men stepped out of the queue and pushed me aside."

Maugham both repeated sounds and blocked. His impediment so demoralized him that, like Philip Carey, the hero of his transparently autobiographical novel *Of Human Bondage,* he evidently lost his faith in God when his prayers for deliverance brought no clear response.

Convinced that a career in politics or the law was beyond his reach, he tried accounting for a while, but eventually decided to become a doctor. In 1897, he qualified as an obstetrician, and published his first novel, *Liza of Lambeth,* based in part on his experiences as an intern. Its modest success encouraged him to abandon medicine, and within a decade he was well established as a writer and financially secure. Indeed, he became a celebrity of sorts and was often sought out for interviews, which he avoided whenever possible, and he refused to give lectures or talks. For the most part, he relied on a succession of private secretaries to handle appointments and other arrangements for him on the phone. This once led to a falling-out he had with D. H. Lawrence, who was offended that Maugham hadn't called himself to arrange a lunch date.

In 1917, Maugham was sent to Russia, ostensibly to write articles on conditions there for the *Daily Telegraph,* but in fact on some sort of clandestine mission to help prop up the Mensheviks. When he was debriefed on his return, he was unable to read his own report, and had to ask his intelligence chief to do it for him.

At the beginning of the Second World War, the British Ministry of Information asked him to travel to the United States as part of a propaganda effort to persuade America to enter the war. He consulted with a speech therapist, who taught him various tricks, such as snapping his fingers hard to break a block, and that gave him confidence enough to proceed. As Maugham rehearsed material for one live interview on NBC radio (from scripts the network writers had worked up), he found it riddled with difficult words, and immediately rewrote the dialogue. As a result, the program went off almost without a hitch. The only trouble came when a brief interlude allowed an impromptu question about who the author of the next great war novel was likely to be. "Well," Maugham replied, "every novelist would rather write about defeat than victory. And j-j-just as the b-b-best novel about the First World War [*All Quiet on the Western Front*] came out of Germany's defeat, so I hope and b-b-b-believe that the best book about this war will come from the same source, and f-f-for the same reason!"

In his later years, Maugham tended to pause and collect himself when he encountered a difficult sound. On his eightieth birthday, he gave a speech at a party thrown in his honor at the Garrick Club. He had learned his speech by heart, and everything went well, apparently,

> until he came to a passage in which he said: "I have reached the stage where I have absorbed all the philosophy I am capable of absorbing and have told all the stories I am able to tell. And I know that anything I may yet have to learn about life will be learned, not from the dusty highways and byways which I frequented in my youth, but from a comparatively secure and certainly more comfortable refuge . . . the v—"
> He stalled at the *v*, and the distinguished assembly sat in silence, staring hypnotized at his lower lip, which desperately sought to make the link with his upper teeth. Instead of giving up in confusion, Maugham stood perfectly still, though his fingers were trembling. After a few moments he said, "I'm just thinking of what I shall say next." Then he lapsed into silence again as ashes dropped from poised cigars and smoke drifted around the ancient pictures. "I'm sorry to keep you waiting," Maugham said, and became silent once more. Then suddenly lip and teeth connected and he came out with it: "the verandah of a luxury hotel."

Psychoanalytical approaches to stuttering tend to be all over the lot, as we have seen, and Maugham has suffered almost as much as Carroll at their hands. One of his biographers suggested that his stutter was "self-inflicted. The stammerer has some quarrel with himself, he sets up his own roadblocks. Stammering becomes a self-fulfilling prophecy." He then conjectures that it was Maugham's "way of punishing himself for the obscure guilt he felt in connection with his mother's death." Without even the pretext of a synoptic bridge, he concludes: "The stammer was a way of telling the world that he was not like others, a way of expressing his singularity. The stammerer is ambivalent about communicating with others—he desperately wants to communicate, but is afraid of revealing himself." Three such very different interpretations have nothing in common with each other except the author's own insecurity about each one. Elsewhere, he identifies the stutter as an appeal for sympathy and says that Maugham substituted a clubfoot for a stammer in *Of Human Bondage* because "a clubfoot is something you are born with, while a stammer is something you do to yourself." The real reason, as Maugham once explained himself, is that it is hard not to make a stutter appear comic in print.

Others have blithely attributed his impediment to severe emotional shock (the death of his mother), a disturbed home life (he grew up in the care of a severe and unsympathetic uncle), nervous self-consciousness, "the sudden demand to speak in a second language" (French was his first), and his homosexuality. It has also been suggested it might have had something to do with an inferiority complex he had about his height, since he "would frequently complain that . . . things would be much different if he were taller." Another biographer states, "Psychologically, the stammerer wants to hold people's attention by withholding the next word," and from this he derives an explanation for Maugham's preference for first-person narration. "He can speak in his own voice—or in the voice he has made us believe is his—without the interruption his stammer so often provided in real life." Anything goes. It may be remembered that one theory claims that stuttering takes place on significant words. The writer Frederick

Prokosch contrarily observed that Maugham "stammered over commonplace words which in their very banality seemed to present some emotional barrier"(!).

One of the therapists who worked with Maugham also worked with King George VI.

Born Albert Frederick Arthur George on December 14, 1895, the future king began to stutter badly at the age of seven or eight, did poorly at school, and in college ranked last in his class. His father berated him for his shortcomings, but that only left him more discouraged than before.

He was an inconspicuous prince, but as he grew to manhood, he inevitably came more into the public eye. Loath to expose his disability, he spurned all interviews and other public functions, and as a naval cadet persuaded a look-alike friend to impersonate him at press conferences and speak on his behalf. On the whole he found it somewhat easier to extemporize than to read from a set text, but much to his family's dismay it was almost impossible for him to say the word "king," as the consonant "k" always stuck in his throat. A number of speech therapists tried to help him, but it wasn't until he was past thirty that one (Lionel Logue) made a difference by teaching him breath control. "He entered my consulting room," Logue later recalled, "at three in the afternoon, a slim, quiet man with tired eyes and all the outward symptoms of the man upon whom habitual speech defect had begun to set the sign." Soon thereafter, the prince optimistically wrote home: "I have been seeing Logue every day, & I have noticed a great improvement in my talking, & also in making speeches which I did this week. I am sure I am going to get quite all right in time, but 24 years of talking in the wrong way cannot be cured in a month. I wish I could have found him before, as now that I know the right way to breathe my fear of talking will vanish."

This represented quite an advance over a few years before when he had awkwardly proposed marriage to Elizabeth (the current Queen Mother) at first through a messenger, and then (when she insisted he do it in person), by handing her a note. When his brother Edward VIII abdicated for love in 1936, it was the last thing George had wanted—"I'm quite unprepared for it," he exclaimed—and we may well believe his biographer that "no monarch ever succeeded more reluctantly to the throne."

Meanwhile, his speech had relapsed completely and Logue was called in to work with him again as he frantically prepared for his coronation speech. Among other things, Logue taught him to interject the syllable "ah" before a particularly troublesome word, and that helped him get through the ceremony without an insurmountable block. However, the annual live Christmas broadcasts he felt obliged to make were "always an ordeal" for him, and he couldn't wait till they were done. One fellow stutterer remembers tuning in with excitement to the first such broadcast he made:

> I got the BBC at the right time and heard, through the static, "Ladies and Gentlemen, His Majesty, King George VI." He started without difficulty, but then his speech began to be more and more labored. He paused between words, first briefly, and then the spaces grew longer. I could sense from the rhythms that a block was coming, and I held my breath waiting for it. There was one long silence, brief sounds of vocal struggle, and then quick repetitions out of which burst the word. This happened several times. . . .

The king worked steadily at controlling his delivery and, over time, gained ground. In his public appearances at least he eventually spoke with relatively little hesitation, particularly toward the end of his life.

Winston Churchill, a most sympathetic witness to the king's ordeals, achieved distinction himself as an orator despite a kind of lisping stutter severe enough to resemble cleft palate speech. From a very early age he engaged in prolonged silent struggles with initial sounds, and (like his father) had particular trouble with the letter "s." With some parental encouragement he used to pace up and down the driveway to his home practicing such sentences as "The Spanish ships I cannot see for they are not in sight." When alliterative exercises failed to help, he consulted with an illustrious throat specialist who assured him that there was nothing physically wrong with his vocal apparatus and that perseverance would prevail.

But as Churchill began to make his way in the world, it did not. Partly as a result of his impediment, he had been a mediocre student, gained admission to the Royal Military College at Sandhurst only on his third try, and upon graduation enlisted in the army, being considered unfit to follow in his father's footsteps with a government career. He saw action in India as a soldier-correspondent, but then in 1899 abruptly resigned his commission to enter politics. His first parliamentary campaign was a disaster, however, and no sooner had the votes been tallied than he sailed for South Africa to report on the Boer War. Soon after he arrived, he participated in a daring operation to rescue an armored train, was captured by the Boers, imprisoned, and escaped. A wanted poster, circulated throughout the Transvaal for his recapture, dead or alive, described him as "about 5' 8" tall;

blonde with a thin light moustache; walks with a slight stoop; cannot speak any Dutch; during long conversations occasionally makes a rattling sound in his throat." Churchill returned to England something of a hero, ran for Parliament again, and narrowly won. But his stump speeches were "painful and embarrassing to listen to," a friend recalled, and an unfavorable review of his maiden speech in Parliament, published in the *Daily Chronicle,* also made note of his hesitant style.

Churchill worked around the problem in his own way. Before attempting to speak, he learned to hum discreetly to himself to get his vocal cords vibrating, and always prepared his remarks with great thoroughness in advance. Indeed, throughout his long and great career he remained quite anxious about the free give-and-take of parliamentary debate, and if suddenly called upon to speak extemporaneously, usually didn't do very well. As Lord Balfour, the longtime Conservative leader once put it, Churchill carried heavy but not very mobile guns. To compensate for exactly this deficiency—that is, not to be caught off guard—he tried to anticipate weeks beforehand the issues that might arise in the House of Commons and the way they would be discussed. He once rather modestly revealed how elaborate his preparations were: "I wrote out my arguments with the greatest care, and then learned them so thoroughly by heart that I knew them backwards and forwards, as well for instance as one knows the Lord's Prayer, and could, within limits, vary the sequence not only of the arguments but of the sentences themselves. . . . Not many people guessed how little spontaneity of conception, fullness of knowledge, or flow of language there was behind this fairly imposing facade."

One of Churchill's prominent political adversaries was

Aneurin Bevan, leader of the left-wing (Bevanite) branch of Britain's Labour Party and the architect of the country's National Health Service plan.

Born in Tredegar, Monmouthshire, in 1897, the son of a miner, he had worked in the collieries as a boy, attended London's Central Labor College, and was elected to the House of Commons in 1929 from Ebbw Vale. Subsequently he served as minister of health in Clement Attlee's Labour government of 1945, and briefly as minister of labor in 1951.

Bevan's speech impediment was remarkably like Churchill's. In addition to a stutter, he had a lisping tendency to make "w's" out of his "r's," and a tendency to get stuck on the letter "s." The problem caused him much pain. "For anyone with a stutter," he once remarked, "the shynesses of youth are magnified out of all proportion." At one point, he consulted the chairman of the South Wales Medical Society, who gave him this advice: "You stammer in speech because you falter in thought. If you can't say it, you don't know it." This had the salutary effect at least of making him more studious, and increasing the care with which he thought his arguments through. As he entered politics, he forced himself to speak as often as possible in public, and did best when his passions were aroused. Yet the trouble remained. "It might be a word beginning with an 's,' " wrote an admirer, "which broke the flow of a beautiful sentence and kept him stammering on the sibilant until he slipped quickly into a synonym and the sentence completed itself." By the age of twenty-five he was able to speak without much hesitation, although his fiery and otherwise effective maiden speech in Parliament was almost spoiled (like Churchill's) by a stuttering block. In time, it is said, "he not so much mastered as brought to life within his personality every skill known to oratory. He knew every gradation of pause and just how long it could be sustained, his gestures were infinite, his sudden use of an exotic word exciting, and he enjoyed a big word along with the scholars. His immense range of inflexion rose and fell like a coloured fountain." In his own day, he was regarded as the best orator in the House of Commons except for Churchill.

Despite their impediments, Churchill and Bevan had become leaders of their country; Nevil Shute, the English novelist and aeronautical engineer, could barely get into the army.

In 1917, when he was eighteen and England at war with Germany, he tried to get a commission in the Royal Engineers, got through his medical examination without stuttering, but upon enrolling in the Royal Military Academy "my officers discovered that on occasion I still stuttered quite a bit." He trained as a gunner for nine months, but by the end of that time, he recalls, "I was stammering very badly from overwork and general war strain, and at my final medical examination I failed and they chucked me out." He underwent three months of speech therapy in an attempt to get back in, but the improvement wasn't enough, so in August of 1918, he enlisted in the infantry. The battalion to which he was assigned, as he soon discovered, was largely made up of men deemed unfit in various ways, and all were posted to extreme rear-guard positions (i.e., in England), as a last line of defense. For the last three months of the war, for example, Shute mounted guard at the mouth of the Thames, even though the Germans "could hardly have invaded us at that stage of the war."

Although he struggled with a lack of self-confidence well into his life, Shute went on to complete his education at

Oxford, became a major innovator in the field of aeronautical design, established a highly successful business around the building of airplanes, and wrote such notable novels as *A Town Like Alice* and *On the Beach*.

Shute regarded his stutter as a symptom of his diffidence. Elizabeth Bowen, the Anglo-Irish novelist and short-story writer, attributed hers to a specific childhood trauma and, her biographer tells us, it "caused her agony as a girl." However,

> it became very much part of her as a woman. It was a stammer, not a stutter—she was very particular about the distinction: stutterers were an altogether different class of person. Elizabeth's stammer was a pronounced hesitation, a complete stalling on certain words. She would help herself out by gestures with her hands, and by substituting a different word. The severity of it varied; it was worse when she was tired, and sometimes almost non-existent when she spoke in public or on television. It did not indicate any lack of confidence in what she was saying; and was often found by others to be an additional charm in her.

A dignified demeanor was of great importance to Bowen; but the distinction she chose to draw between stammering and stuttering, which favored her own particular form of the affliction, is without moral meaning, and clinically profitless. There is nothing inherently more dignified about one kind of involuntary muscular spasm than another, although repetitions may seem more disorderly than blocks.

That being said, her own pride and determined efforts at self-control probably helped her. Although unwilling to act in a play, for example, she did lecture successfully, and among sympathetic friends at least her witty conversation flowed with ease. V. S. Pritchett described her impediment as a "lovely whistling stammer," and her lover, the Canadian diplomat Charles Ritchie, adoringly remarked on "the stammering flow of her enthralling talk." She herself wasn't quite so enamored of it, and although she sat on a number of committees was anxious enough about faltering to rarely say a word. On her deathbed, however, according to her biographer, her stammer "completely disappeared."

A stutter can sometimes be such an obstacle to free expression that, given the inclination, it may act as a powerful incentive to write. In the case of Edward Hoagland his "vocal handcuffs," as he called them, ultimately led him to favor the personal essay as "the closest thing to speech."

In his youth Hoagland had made a number of discouraging ventures into therapy, beginning at age eleven, when his parents took him to a speech pathologist. She taught him to put one hand in his pocket and write over and over again the first letter of the word he was trying to pronounce. This worked briefly, but proved "more unsettling to other people than the ailment it was meant to cure." So at fifteen he was sent to a speech camp in Michigan where (under threat of corporal punishment) he was taught to speak so slowly "that it didn't seem like speech at all." Later, at Harvard, he tried therapy of the Iowa school—deliberate stuttering and seeking out situations that even a normal speaker might avoid: for example, accosting authority figures or strangers on the street. He found this exercise in conditioning quite useless. But such was his social handicap, as he candidly explained, that the loss of his virginity was delayed until he met a woman willing "to take command" and make "the verbal preliminaries unnecessary."

In his stories he shows himself particularly sympathetic to

down-and-out characters and to those whom life has dealt a poor hand. His tender love of animals, which permeates his work, is also, he believes, bound up with his speech because human communication was so hard.

In the face of such a medical conundrum, as we have seen, everyone (including the afflicted) has been more or less free to conjecture about it as they pleased. One of Charles I's biographers, for example, tells us that his impediment was "probably the symptom of some boiling subterranean rage." Another, unable to decide, hedges his bets: "Heredity, prenatal disturbance, childhood worries, the anxiety of physical infirmity, all could have played their part." In the end he inclines to the view that Charles was probably scared out of his wits by gory nursery tales. In the case of George VI, it was thought by some that he developed his stutter because of a forced shift in handedness; others tied it to hostility toward his father, who looked upon him with such a disapproving eye. Aneurin Bevan had an uncle who stuttered, and his mother thought he had caught it by mimicry or imitation. Robert Boyle subscribed to the same idea. Charles Darwin, on the other hand, believed that stuttering was inherited because, of course, it ran in his family. Somerset Maugham rather late in life met a stuttering relation and surmised it must be in his genes. Erasmus Darwin faulted his own vanity and desire to show off; Cotton Mather factored in his sins; Leigh Hunt blamed his physical frailty and an overprotective mother; Margaret Drabble attributed Arnold Bennett's impediment to a tyrannical father. Oddly expanding on this idea, she connected it with an "over-rigorous pot-training which Arnold like all his generation probably suffered from." If so, then we should expect most middle-to-late Victorians to have speech defects. Bennett himself thought it had something to do with conflicting (or conflicted) thoughts. Clara Barton found the cause in her childhood terrors, Moses Mendelssohn in an overactive mind, Elizabeth Bowen in the spectacle of her father's mental breakdown, Marilyn Monroe in being sexually abused as a child. John Updike apparently accepts Wendell Johnson's diagnosogenic theory—though unable to recall any instance of parental overcorrection from his own formative years.

The biblical prophet Moses, as a man of suprahistorical destiny, in the end can only have seen in his impediment the all-knowing and infinite purpose of God.

In whatever way the disorder has been understood, most of the notable people described—like anonymous sufferers everywhere—have managed to cope with some measure of success. Demosthenes, George VI, and John Updike, for example, seem to have benefited most from breath control; Charles I, Lewis Carroll, Winston Churchill, and Aneurin Bevan found it helpful to know exactly what they were going to say in advance; Churchill got his vocal cords vibrating as a warmup; Charles I also learned something from the continuous phonation of song; Robert Boyle and Cotton Mather both spoke in an extremely slow and deliberate fashion; Erasmus Darwin methodically practiced on initial sounds; Charles Lamb eased his self-consciousness a bit by drinking; Charles Kingsley distracted himself by putting a piece of cork between his teeth; Clara Barton stabilized her articulators; perhaps the roaring waves of the sea helped Demosthenes concentrate by drowning out the sound of his own voice; and so on. All, in a sense, had a piece of the puzzle. Yet nothing entire.

# Part Three

## Deliverance

# Chapter Seven

"The aim should be, not the cure of stammering, but the development of correct speech. . . . [The stammerer] must be taught to bring all the processes of speech within the domain of his own consciousness, and he must learn to control them by volitional effort in the manner of a musician learning to play upon a violin."

—G. HUDSON MAKUEN, *Professor of Defects of Speech at the University of Pennsylvania, 1931*

As far as I know, I began to stutter at about the age of eight—at least I first became conscious of my stutter at that time. As everyone develops their own theory as to where their stutter comes from, mine was that it was somehow connected to my mother's death. She had stuttered, and so I later wondered if I had incorporated her impediment into myself as a way of holding on to some part of her once she was gone. This may seem overingenious, but it made the more sense to me because, as it happens, she had also taught me how to spell. It was only as an adult that it occurred to me that, since my eldest brother stutters too, it was highly unlikely that we both would have adopted the same curious psychic stratagem.

My brother's stutter was always rather mild; mine was pronounced, and included a tendency to "block" or stop dead on certain sounds. My mouth would open, but no voice emerge. I went through school trying to say as little in class as I could, and used all the avoidance behaviors I have ever heard of to conceal the terrible secret of my inability to speak. I became an adept at word substitution, clever at paraphrase, and an ambulatory thesaurus of synonyms as a means to help me evade "difficult" sounds. I also cultivated a brief, reserved, even abrupt manner of speech (interspersed with many "thoughtful" hesitations), and in this way succeeded pretty well at times with my masquerade.

Nevertheless, I always knew myself to be handicapped. Each day I would set forth determined, as if my life depended on it, to slay this dragon, only to find that my speech had a life of its own. My overriding purpose from about the age of ten was, in every situation involving contact with another human soul, to somehow not make a fool of myself—though in one way or another, of course, that happened all the time.

Moreover, although decidedly expert at mannerisms of avoidance and a covert stutterer to a high degree, I was nevertheless among those comparatively rare individuals who stuttered even when reading aloud to themselves.

By the time I entered college, I felt better able to manage

in informal settings, and wondered briefly if, by some strange luck, I might actually "outgrow" my mysterious malady. Yet in retrospect it seems to me that I wasn't so much better as more of an adept. Besides, I had reached an age when I could drink, and I found, frankly, that that helped me to relax. And of course I continued to avoid stuttering situations when I could. Classroom participation was seldom obligatory; but seminars were a trial. There I contrived to contribute by overlapping my comments onto the conclusion of what someone else said. This had to be done carefully so as not to seem rude or to interrupt, but when it worked the sound of their voice fading covered my own initial hesitations and gave me confidence to proceed. Days of reckoning, however, always come. I remember (with embarrassment), for example, being asked by my Chaucer professor to read aloud an essay I had written on "The Franklin's Tale" to the class. For me, that was out of the question, and I contrived to be ill over the next few weeks until discussion of that part of Chaucer's work was safely past.

I persevered. After I dropped out of school abruptly in the middle of my sophomore year (basically, I had a nervous breakdown), I returned a year later, and graduated from Columbia College in the winter of 1971, with a Kellett fellowship to Oxford. Columbia also offered me a graduate fellowship, and I stayed. In the following year, I earned my Master's Degree in English and Comparative Literature, and began to look down the road toward my doctoral orals a couple of years away. Time came; time went: the day drew near. When it finally arrived, I hid my terror as best I could behind some extremely eccentric verbal behavior and clouds of cigarette smoke. Actually, by the time I walked into the room I was almost as worried about having a heart attack as I was about my speech. For weeks I had lived on brandy and cigarettes, and for three nights running had been virtually unable to sleep. I think my examiners must have been mystified since I'd had no trouble at all with the pre-oral written exam. All I can remember now of my performance is that I let everybody down. Thanks to the magnanimity of the examiners, I passed, but shortly thereafter I left school, convinced no teaching career could ever be for me. Subsequently, I took a number of odd jobs—as leathercraftsman, file clerk, book binder, book production assistant, and so on—often at salaries not much above minimum wage. In truth, I felt myself unfit for anything else.

A complete sense of worthlessness and failure overcame me, and a profound depression. I had no sense of capacity or achievement, and (such is speech to our sense of self) regarded myself simply as a stutterer, fundamentally inadequate at life.

When I married, my wife and I started a music-management business together (she was musical; I contributed the graphic design), and this seemed to hold out the possibility to me of an independent and adequate livelihood. Nevertheless, I had nothing to do with the phone work, and dreaded the terrible awkwardness that resulted whenever I had to field a call. Meanwhile, from 1979 to 1980, I worked on my first book, *Labyrinths of Iron,* at night. It was published in 1981, and graciously received; but I was unable to take advantage of the interview opportunities that arose. When I subsequently decided to write a biography of Russia's first tsar (as a way of exploring Russian life at the height of the Renaissance in the West), I called my agent but couldn't pronounce "Ivan the Terrible" on the phone. He patiently ran down a random list of the tsars, and when he came to Ivan I said, "Thank you, yes."

That pathetic episode was not unrepresentative of what, each day, I faced. Some stutterers find that liquor aggravates their impediment; I did not. But I drank more than was required. My dependency found its way into some of the epigrams I was writing—and though these were not "confessional" in genre, they nevertheless reflected (like my poem on Caedmon) realities of my life. I retain a fondness for a few of them, including one "On Craft & Inspiration," which seems to me now (beyond its own self-bemusement) to capture something of my world in brief:

> For every four-line epigram I write,
> I scotch four lines at least to get it tight.
> It takes a fifth of Scotch to get it right.

The truth is, I drank pretty much anything that came to hand. And the gradual erosion of my marriage was not unconnected to these strains.

Although unforgiving toward anyone who showed the least impatience with my speech, the lover of the English language in me could still sympathize with John Marston's otherwise harsh Elizabethan diatribe against "the vildest stumbling stutterer that ever hack'd and hew'd our native tongue." At one time or another over the years I had seen a speech pathologist, a hypnotist, and a psychotherapist. None of them had done me any good. Then one day in the spring of 1986, I happened to watch a movie on one of the new cable channels I had just hooked up called *Talk to Me*, which dramatized a relatively new therapy developed by Ronald L.

Webster at the Hollins Communications Research Institute in Roanoke, Virginia.

The star of the movie was Austin Pendleton, the distinguished actor and director, who had once remarked (as a stutterer) that he had gone into acting "with the same impulse that drives cripples to become athletes." Not inappropriately, he had first appeared on Broadway as Jonathan the stutterer in Arthur Kopit's play *Oh Dad, Poor Dad, Mama's Hung You in the Closet and I'm Feelin' So Sad.* "Never again," he later vowed in an interview, "will I play the part of a stutterer. It's hard enough to control anyway. When you're acting one, you're in the lap of the gods every night." (In fact, not only did he subsequently recapitulate such a role, brilliantly, in *Talk to Me,* but more recently appeared as the stuttering lawyer in the movie *My Cousin Vinny.*)

Although Pendleton found he could manage onstage, offstage he couldn't say his credit card number on the telephone. "By the time I was 40," he recalled, "stuttering was driving me crazy. I was exhausting myself out of nervousness, not expressing what I really wanted to say. More than one theater critic said they liked my performance, but without my stutter I could really have been brilliant. In the movie, *The First Family,* I really had trouble saying my lines." One day in 1981, when he was directing Elizabeth Taylor and Maureen Stapleton in *The Little Foxes* on Broadway, he accidentally came upon an article that recounted the ordeals of Annie Glenn.

Anyone who has read Tom Wolfe's *The Right Stuff* is likely to remember the scene where Annie Glenn (wife of the astronaut and longtime Ohio senator) refused to talk to Vice President Lyndon Johnson on national TV. On January 27, 1962, as the countdown had begun at Cape Canaveral for her husband's lift-off into space, she frantically paced back and forth in her living room, her terror of stammering before the entire nation exceeding her anxiety about the impending launch. Johnson kept clamoring to get in; but she kept the door barred.

As a child she had stuttered on just about every word, and not much amelioration had come with time. Like a deaf-mute, she used to write out her destination for bus and taxi drivers, and in restaurants order by number or point to the item on the menu she desired. Sometimes she would just order whatever she could say, even if it wasn't what she wanted to eat. In stores, she would look in vain for merchandise rather than ask a clerk for help. Her husband had to make the calls to friends and repairmen; her neighbors were depended upon to call the doctor if her children became ill.

It was the highly publicized and successful therapy that Annie Glenn underwent, followed by Austin Pendleton and others, that called attention to an approach that eventually led to my own deliverance.

Ronald Webster's therapy had emerged from some remarkable new scientific developments. One formative event is nicely recounted by speech pathologist Oliver Bloodstein:

> One day in or around 1950, an electronic engineer with the Signal Corps at Fort Monmouth, Bernard S. Lee, was trying out a new, state-of-the-art tape recorder by recording his own voice. Included in the equipment was a set of headphones through which the operator could listen to a recording as it was being made. By error, Lee had plugged the headphones into the wrong jack. Through a peculiarity in the design of the device, this caused him to hear his

recorded speech with a slight delay in transmission, so that everything he heard in the headphones was what he had said a fraction of a second before. Under these conditions Lee, who is a normal speaker, found to his surprise that he was involuntarily repeating the first syllables of words. He was so intrigued by this effect, that he wrote an article entitled "Artificial Stutter" and sent it to the Journal of Speech and Hearing Disorders, where it was published in 1951.

When others were subjected to the same delayed feedback, they either repeated syllables like Lee, or spontaneously prolonged them in an effort to slow their speech down. This led to speculation that the auditory feedback system of the stutterer might be impaired in some analogous way. Subsequently it was also discovered that when a stutterer was subjected to high-frequency white noise above eighty-five decibels in both ears (loud enough to mask the sound of his own voice), his fluency improved. The conclusions to be drawn were these: if being unable to hear your own voice helped, then perhaps hearing it was part of the problem; and the nature of the problem appeared (from Lee's discovery) to involve the auditory feedback loop.

The "feedback" concept derives from cybernetics, a term coined in 1948 for the comparative study of automatic control systems in which errors in the output are returned to the source so that corrections can be made. The familiar mechanical-electrical model was inspired by biology, for all creatures instantaneously regulate their physical actions by comparing them, through various mechanisms, with what they were intended to be. Auditory feedback through the ear, for example, informs the speaker about the pitch, volume, and inflection of his voice, the accuracy of articulation, selection of the appropriate words, and so forth. Another feedback system, involving sensory structures within the muscles, tendons, and joints, provides continual information as to their position, movement, and feel.

It had long been known that speech and hearing were connected. Stuttering is uncommon among the deaf and severe hard-of-hearing, and a child born deaf does not normally progress in speech beyond the "babbling" stage. A child needs to hear the sounds he will learn to make—to hear how others make them, and how he makes them himself. In this way he learns to associate sounds with the vocal movements that produce them. And by hearing he makes the adjustments in voice and articulation that the language of his environment requires. Although it wasn't until recently that it occurred to anyone that the way in which a stutterer hears his own voice (or doesn't hear it) might have something to do with his infirmity, in retrospect information concerning the deaf provided clues.

But riddling problems remained. First, it was apparent that the stutter-like speech elicited from a normal speaker under conditions of artificial delay was not stuttering in the clinical sense. Prolongations occurred in the middle of words, and repetitions at the end, whereas almost all real stuttering occurs on initial sounds; moreover, when stutterers were subjected to Lee's experiment, to everyone's astonishment, they became more fluent, as their speech became more purposeful and slow.

Well before this phenomenon could be fully understood, clinicians seized upon it as a therapeutic tool. Since the duration of the delay determined the rate of speech, it was used to oblige stutterers to speak at the slowest possible rate as a foundation for applying other remedial techniques.

While tantalizing questions were being explored with regard to the auditory feedback loop, other discoveries about the physiology of the stutterer were being made.

This process began in the 1930s—about the time, that is, that the "neurotic tendencies" or "personality peculiarities" of stutterers were being catalogued. In subsequent years, they were subjected to Fear Survey Schedules, the Palmar Sweat Index (a physiologic measure of negative emotion), blood, brain wave, and dichotic listening tests, reaction time studies, and so on; and in addition to obvious signs of tension (like tremors), it was found that in the anticipation and moment of stuttering, abnormal changes took place: in breathing, heart and pulse rate, blood composition (as manifested by a drop in blood sugar and protein), and blood distribution. There was also increased electrical skin conductance, the pupils of the eyes were found to dilate, and odd brain wave patterns showed up on electroencephalograms. Using magnetic resonance imaging and radioactive tracers absorbed into the blood, researchers also found subtle irregularities in hemispheric blood flow and digital volume during speech. At first it was thought, as Van Riper put it, that these were "probably no more than the reflection of the stress [the stutterer] feels. They are the physiologic correlates of his struggle or fear."

But as other evidence accumulated, more might be said. For example, overall lags in simple motor coordination and speech reaction times showed up, indicating a fundamental problem with central nervous system function. While the problem might not be great enough to prevent excellence at sports (as Bob Love, Lester Hayes, Ken Venturi, and other athletic stars amply prove), the least disruption in the system's subtle integration would, if anywhere, be reflected in speech, the most finely tuned of all motor skills. Moreover, electromyographic data and fiber-optic films revealed abnormally high tension levels in the laryngeal speech muscles and distorted activity of the vocal folds whether stuttering occurred or not. Even during episodes of seemingly perfect fluency, a faint crackling sound could still be detected, indicating that the voicing was not functionally relaxed. At such moments, the rules of speech mechanics were still being broken, and the speaker by a kind of transient luck was just coasting above the breaking point.

At the very least, all this suggested, in one assessment, "a need for the stutterer to take more time to coordinate the complexities of the speech act." But the larger lesson seemed to be that fear reduction, deliberate stuttering, and other such desensitizing strategies would never be adequate: in the end, the stutterer would have to learn how to voice and articulate correctly, or (no matter how self-accepting he might be) he would always remain on the threshold of verbal disintegration. He would always be skating on thin ice.

Meanwhile, genetic studies had begun to provide a second tier of evidence that the disorder was physically based. By the mid-1970s, it had been determined, for example, that immediate relatives were three times more likely to stutter than those at some remove, with male relatives of female stutterers at greatest risk. The co-twin of a stuttering monozygotic (identical) twin had a 77 percent chance of stuttering; the co-twin of a dizygotic (fraternal) twin a 32 percent chance; the ordinary sibling of a stutterer a 20 percent chance. Moreover, 54 percent of the children of mothers who stuttered and 24 percent of afflicted fathers stuttered themselves. While this hereditary pattern did not correspond to the classic Mendelian paradigms explaining the recurrence of physical traits, it did indicate an inherited neurologic susceptibility, such as might also explain the incidence of disorders like dyslexia, dysgraphia, or Gilles de la Tourette syndrome.

By contrast, nongenetic patterns of transmission failed to hold up under scrutiny. Stuttering was found to occur among siblings without respect to birth, rank, or age separation, and children separated at birth from an afflicted parent or sibling were just as likely to develop a stutter as those who were not. Imitation, therefore, could not play a significant role. Nor could environment, however much it might aggravate the disorder once it appeared. Throughout the world, the average age of onset, incidence, and male-to-female ratio of the affliction (which itself indicated a sex-linked gene) was proving to be about the same.

A third tier of developing evidence was pharmacological. Drug therapy of one sort or another, of course, had been around since ancient times, and in the late nineteenth century, sedatives such as tincture of peppermint oil and chloroform had been administered to calm spasms of the diaphragm. In the 1940s, carbon dioxide was experimentally tried, when it was also used to treat phobic disorders and dissociative states. More recent medications—Bellergal-S, hydroxyzine (an antihistamine with sedative properties), tranquilizers like reserpine and meprobamate, and (in Russia) bromides combined with calcium chloride—have targeted secondary symptoms of stuttering, like anxiety and stress. Thiamine and other vitamin supplements have also been prescribed (as relaxants), as has verapamil, a blood pressure medicine that controls muscle contractions. However, only the neuroleptic drug haloperidol had any demonstrable effect. As it happens, haloperidol also alleviates the symptoms of Tourette's syndrome by means of dopamine receptor and calcium blocking activity.

In short, all signs had begun to point to a developmental disorder of the central nervous system, "possibly derived," as one expert put it, "from subtle abnormalities of central auditory functioning or sensory motor-processing."

Centuries of sometimes arbitrary theorizing seemed at last to be hastening to an end. In a fundamental paper on the subject entitled "The Establishment of Fluent Speech in Stutterers," presented at the American Association for the Advancement of Tension Control in London in September 1979, Ronald Webster summarized the new empirical evidence and, on the basis of it, the conclusions to be drawn. These (and they bear repeating) included: that stuttering is a physically based problem; that it tends to run in families, whether or not the affected members are known to each other at first hand; and that a tendency to the disorder, if not the disorder itself, is inherited, as evidenced by the fact, that (1) it occurs throughout the world in all language groups, with an incidence of about 1 percent; (2) the developmental course of the disorder is universally consistent, with about 95 percent of all cases occurring by the age of seven; and (3) the sex ratio of the disorder, which affects four times as many males as females, is also consistent worldwide. Adopting the cybernetic paradigm (according to which there is an abrupt increase in the level of a system's output when a feedback signal is disrupted), Webster pointed out that the repetitions, prolongations, and blockings characteristic of stuttered speech all represented forms of "overshooting" in that the muscle movements involved were made with undue force. As correlative evidence that disturbed auditory feedback was somehow implicated, he noted that most of the ways in which fluency is enhanced—by whispering, singing, or choral reading, and under conditions of auditory feedback and white noise masking—had their "loci of effects at either the larynx or the ear." He therefore concluded that stuttering was essentially "a motor control disorder," and that the probable mechanism responsible was a defect in the auditory feedback loop.

An experimental psychologist with degrees from the University of Maine and Louisiana State University, Webster had been working on the problem of stuttering since 1966. Originally concerned with speech and language development in infants—in particular, with how the sounds a baby hears influence the sounds he is making—he turned his attention to stuttering as a result of questions raised by a colleague. He reviewed the current status of therapeutic theory and practice, found it unsatisfactory from a scientific point of view, and began to look for scientific facts that were replicable in designing an objective approach. He took note of the delayed auditory feedback experiments that had recently been conducted, tried operant conditioning (reward and punishment), relaxation therapy (to determine if anxiety was at the heart of the problem), and even the power of positive thinking, without appreciable success. Meanwhile, he had also been experimenting with physical behaviors such as sound and syllable prolongation, variations in the amplitude and speed of voicing and articulation, breathing, and so on, and by 1974, through computer analysis, speech spectrography, and other electronic measurement techniques, had been able to identify "a series of tiny but absolutely critical speech movement characteristics" that appeared to be precursors to fluent speech. These were precisely and empirically defined and incorporated into several muscle movement patterns, or "targets," which became the basis for the now-famous Hollins "Precision Fluency Shaping Program."

"For a stutterer to speak fluently," Webster noted, "the movements of speech must be held within certain limits of rate and force." To begin with, speech was therefore drastically slowed, and with the help of a stopwatch the duration of each syllable, and each sound within the syllable, was uniformly "stretched." Once "slow motion speech" had been established, it became possible to isolate, and then deliberately change, distorted speech behaviors that could not otherwise be identified when speech occurred at a normal rate. Upon that foundation, over the course of one hundred twenty hours of intensive practice the stutterer could learn how to stabilize his articulators for initial sound positions; manage soft articulatory contact on consonants; properly complete the articulatory gestures for ending syllables; acquire control over diaphragmatic breathing (the basis for voice onset training); and establish correct control over the laryngeal muscles responsible for the production of voice.

To help teach precise control over voice onsets and their coordination with articulation, Webster invented a small, fixed-purpose, radio-size computer, called a Voice Monitor, that measured voice amplitude at the beginning of an utterance and its rate of increase or "intensity rise time." Its maddeningly precise reaction may be deemed indispensable, for the Gentle Onset Target, as it is called (and the fundamental target of the program), is extremely difficult to get right. Almost all voice blockages occur on hard onsets, when in attempting any vowel or consonant sound, the vocal folds are closed too abruptly and the breath stream is initiated with too much force. When, on the other hand, voicing is natural, it involves gentle, low-amplitude vocal fold vibrations that gradually increase in strength, then decrease to the initial level before the articulation of a following sound. The pattern of such vibrations forms a "loudness contour" that may be pictured as a kind of bell curve.

Other targets involved reducing excessive air pressure in the vocal tract (with voiceless fricatives like "f" or "s" or plusive consonants like "b" or "d"), and effecting smooth transitions from one sound to another (for example, from "m" to "o"), since the speech mechanism, as Webster observes, does not operate the way a typewriter does when you type a word, by making isolated sounds, but is actually in the process of beginning the next sound while the first is being produced. Once the targets have been mastered, sounds are combined into words, words into phrases, and the rate of speech is gradually increased. The newly acquired skills are transferred from the clinic to outside settings, and the therapy is complete.

All the targets, however, must be understood not only in concept, but "at the level of muscle activity." And so they must be sustained. When practiced repeatedly, they not only retrain the speech musculature, but enable the stutterer, through tactile and proprioceptive feedback, to acquire the true *feel* of correct speech. By that feel *(not by hearing, which may be faulty)* he can more accurately monitor his speech production.

The kinesthetic feedback system is quicker and more reliable anyway, as one therapist points out—"You know if it's right or not in the moment that it's happening. But to hear it you have to say it, and by then it's too late. At that point you're hearing it again in your mind and asking yourself, 'Was that right?' "

It would be utterly futile of course to try to consciously manage a serially ordered motor activity without some way of precisely tracking the muscle movements involved. And it would be particularly futile to try to do so by thought rather than feel. That is why the most enlightened attempts by earlier theorists, such as Erasmus Darwin, Warren, Combe, Voisin, Hunt, Makuen, and others to develop a therapeutic program for conscious speaking failed. For centuries stutterer and therapist alike had had to content themselves with relatively vague and impressionistic notions of what was required—to speak more slowly, breathe more naturally, keep the vocal cords vibrating, and so on; but for a neuromuscular coordination as subtle as speech, such notions were far too vague to suffice.

It may be remembered that Wendell Johnson told his clients, "Stuttering is not something that happens to you. It is something that you do." Webster turned it around: "When you entered this program," he would often remind those at the end of it, "your speech *was* something that happened to you. Specifically, stuttering happened to you. Now you are responsible for your own speech."

There are many other therapies to be had, of course—some resembling Webster's, and drawing on the same general empirical data; some not. But this was the therapy that worked for me. Though skeptical that any therapy could, in mid-April 1986 I called the Hollins Institute to enroll, only to be told that no openings would be available until the following year. I subsequently learned that the Communications Reconstruction Center, a speech therapy clinic in New York, used the same approach. I went in to see the head clinician there, Catherine Otto, who interviewed me at length, variously assessed my speech, and diagnosed me as a "moderate to moderately severe stutterer." She had an opening in a summer program, and I took it: that was eight years ago, and I have seldom stuttered since.

In 1987, the year after I completed my therapy, my biography of Ivan the Terrible (*Fearful Majesty*), was published, offered as a Main Selection of the History Book Club, and led to interview requests that I was now prepared to oblige. Fluency, however (as an acquired skill), can never be taken for granted, and no occasion for speech is without challenges that must be faced. For a stutterer (even one reformed like myself) that is just the way it is. Nevertheless, a regular routine of formal practice, or a solitary review for about twenty minutes each day of what correct speech requires, seems to be enough to keep the musculature primed.

In light of the new evidence, many old assumptions will have to go. It is still axiomatic in the clinical literature, for example, that speech is facilitated by "distraction." In the case of an odd accent or vocal posturing, peculiar body movement, and so on, this may be so; but "distraction" has also been invoked to explain fluency in whispering, choral reading, reading in unison, singing, even white noise masking and delayed auditory feedback. Upon examination, distraction would seem to have little to do with any of these.

It is a feature of any distraction that its effectiveness diminishes with time. However, speakers seem not to adapt to white noise masking, rhythm, or auditory feedback; and in choral reading the stutterer is not distracted from, but rather has to concentrate on, synchronizing his speech with other members of the group. In singing, the speaker likewise has to synchronize his speech to music (even as the music helps him to pattern his speech in time). Again, delayed auditory feedback requires him to slow his speech down; whispering, to enunciate slowly and with care. In fact, the ameliorative effect of all these ways of "speaking" is best explained by the hypothesis that they eliminate or compensate in some way for a disturbance in the auditory feedback loop. And they do this in general by obliging the speaker to assume greater control over the speech act. The one exception proves the rule: in white noise masking, there is no disturbance, because there is no auditory self-perception at all.

In keeping with the shift from mouth to ear, most appliances designed today to help the stutterer typically resemble a hearing aid. One is an electronic metronome with a rhythmic tick to help in the pacing of speech; another drowns out the speaker's own vocal feedback by means of white noise; a third (developed by Webster) amplifies the sound of phonation by means of a tiny microphone placed just behind the earlobe where the jaw and skull are joined. In this way (somewhat circumventing the auditory feedback loop), the sound is delivered "directly" to the ear. Known as the "Fluency Master," Webster's device has recently been adopted by the Mayo Clinic and is the centerpiece of the stuttering therapy program at the William Beaumont Hospital in Detroit.

We hear our own speech, of course, in two different ways—through air conduction (with about a twenty millisecond delay) from mouth to ear, as we hear the speech of another; and by resonance through the bone and tissue of the skull. By resonance, I mean the underlying sound of our phonation (the vibrations of our vocal cords) as conveyed from the larynx to the inner ear. The first is articulated speech, the second its foundation, an inarticulate moan. That's why our voice sounds different to us on tape.

Webster's original hypothesis (formulated in 1974) about the cause of the disorder centered on two tiny middle ear muscles known as the tensor tympani and the stapedius, which are neurologically coordinated with the larynx and which contract a fraction of a second before the start of phonation to protect the inner ear from the blast of one's own voice. He surmised that in stutterers their contraction instead occurred simultaneously with phonation, so that the signal of voice was returned out of sync to the brain. This was borne out with respect to stuttered speech, but not to a stutterer's fluent productions.

Webster next directed his attention to the nature of sound transmission through the skull, where studies of phase disparities between air- and bone-conducted tones indicated strongly that there was an apparent distortion, phase shift, or lag in a signal passing through the stutterer's skull. "If we vibrate the skull of the stutterer with a tunable oscillator," he explained recently,

> at about the same frequency with which the vocal folds are opening and closing, we generate fluent speech. But if we vibrate the skull at a frequency somewhat removed from the basic vibrational read of the voice, we don't. So there may be some critical skull resonance characteristics involved in disturbing the normal return of sensory information to the

brain. We're talking here about the very structure of the skull: the configuration, the mass, the coupling of skull plates, the coupling of the skull to the cartilage and soft tissue of the neck region, the larynx—the whole energy transfer system.

Webster's resonance theory may ultimately explain the riddle of fluent whispering—because in whispering there is no resonance, since phonation has been turned off.

Research continues, in this and other areas; but whatever the conflicting views, few doubt today that stuttering is an inheritable, physically based disorder. The real scientific debate has to do with the precise neurological or language processing function involved. Although it is still not completely clear what the brain does to facilitate speech, it is known that both cerebral hemispheres are involved in processing language, though in different capacities. The left (in normal right-handers) is involved in speech production, but is also able to analyze the constituent parts of sentences and process verbs and nouns; the right is better able to process high-imagery nouns and adjectives, or associative and connotative meanings. The first ("Broca's area") is involved with the motor elaboration of all the movements for expressive language; the second ("Wernicke's area"), receptive speech comprehension. Although the difference in which these language centers operate is still being explored, shift of handedness has been shown to have no appreciable impact on speech. The incidence of stuttering among children who break or otherwise lose the use of an arm does not increase, nor has it been found to be greater among people with one arm. On the other hand, recent evidence seems to justify speculation as to some compensatory overinvolvement in stutterers of the brain's right hemisphere in speech, possibly "because of a maturational delay in left hemisphere development or of some physical dysfunction at the level of the thalamus or lower brain-stem." It has also been suggested that stuttering may originate in the left supplementary motor area of the brain, with reference to the organization and initiation of speech sounds. Still other research similarly implies a dysfunction in the phonological encoding process involved in speech planning. According to this theory, stuttering results from trying to speak before the articulatory plan of the utterance has been specified in the brain.

All such speculation shares in the notion that there is something wrong with the neurological wiring involved. Moreover, while a definitive cure remains elusive, there are now techniques that have produced successful results. Nevertheless, the ranks of speech pathologists remain split on philosophical grounds. At least since the mid-1930s, in fact, therapists have divided themselves into the so-called "speak differently" and "stutter differently" camps. Webster obviously belongs to the former; generally speaking, those under the influence (or within the tradition) of Van Riper and Johnson belong to the latter. Bloodstein recently summed up the difference between the two: "Methods that teach stutterers to talk differently almost always result in fluency at the cost of the necessity to monitor speech, some unnaturalness, and vulnerability to relapse. Methods that teach people to stutter differently allow them to speak naturally with no special attention to their speech (except when they stutter), and generally don't leave them helpless in relapse. The cost is the abandonment of any aspiration to speak with normal fluency."

I have my own bias, of course, and so for a moment enter the discussion as a partisan. It may be doubted, to begin with, that any (uncorrected) utterance by a stutterer can be considered "natural" (in light of what we now know about the physiology of it), while modifications like the slide or the bounce are themselves "talk differently" approaches, since their aim is to control the stutterer's speech. Nor in fairness can it be said that a program such as Webster's leaves the speaker "helpless in relapse," since the conscientious practitioner can always return to the techniques he has learned. The time and effort it takes to learn how to stutter effortlessly (whatever that may mean) might, perhaps, be better spent learning how to speak naturally, or correctly, in the physiological sense. After all, if you're going to go down the road of speech modification, you might as well expend your energy on a form of modification that leads to fluent speech. To accept yourself as a stutterer can also mean to accept what, as a stutterer, you have to do to speak correctly. There is no "false role" in that.

That being said, I do appreciate (and know, from my own experience) that this controversy has another, subtler side. One contributor to *Letting Go*, the newsletter of the National Stuttering Project, put it well:

Why did fluency controls never become habitual or automatic? I think the answer lies in the nature of the way that speech operates. Everything about it functions automatically, that is, the formulation of ideas, the generation of sentences, of phrases, of words, of sounds. . . . Working memory seems to have a finite capacity at any given time. To the extent that this capacity is taxed by attention to the motor skills that promote fluency, it is thereby unavailable for attention to the communication of ideas. To expect people who stutter to maintain controlled fluency day in and day out for extended periods is to expect them to abandon the way the speaking system was designed to operate.

John Harrison, an editor of the newsletter, may have glimpsed the answer when he wrote: "At some point, like the Zen archer, you must stop *trying* to shoot the arrow correctly, and get out of your own way."

The problem is not really one of monitoring—after all, an archer who neglects to practice will eventually find he can't even bend his bow—but of a state of mind. Some stutterers, for example, are unable to take full advantage of physical therapy because they remain "speech doubters"—unable to take that necessary leap of faith into believing in their own ability to speak. And here, I think, the anticipatory struggle hypothesis stands on solid ground—not as a pathogenic explanation of stuttering, but as an indispensable component of successful therapy. In therapy and beyond, a willing suspension of disbelief is required to avoid relapses from therapeutic gains. Two main factors (I would venture) lead to relapse. The first is that the stutterer, either through lack of practice, or lack of proper attention during practice, loses the ability to discriminate the subtle muscle movement details. The second is a lack of confidence, a kind of fatalism really, bred in him by countless episodes of defeat, that the skill itself won't work. There is no doubt that even a touch of self-consciousness, especially when it is in the least apprehensive, will tend to throw speech off. Scanning ahead and anticipating trouble is often the last of the vicious habits to disappear—and the first to reassert itself with any faltering sound. Vocal faith enables the speaker to concentrate properly, without undue effort, on the speech mechanics he has learned. In effect, it allows speech to be more or less automatic, even as its flow is governed by a continuous feel. Anxiety, on the other hand, results in too little—or too much—monitoring, and begins to break speech down.

The idea of excessive monitoring was once amusingly described by one beleaguered stutterer who drew an analogy between his own predicament and that of the storied centipede who ran happily along

> . . . until the frog in fun
> Said, "Pray, which leg comes after which?"
> This raised his mind to such a pitch,
> He lay distracted in the ditch,
> Considering how to run.

No image could be more appropriate—or numerically right, given the hundred odd muscles involved in the coordination of simple speech. At the same time, I am reminded of Heinrich von Kleist's famous meditation "On the Puppet Theater," in which two men have a remarkable conversation about the nature of graceful movement in dance. One of the two, a famous dancer himself, explains the manipulation of the puppets to his companion:

> "Each movement," he said, "had its center of gravity; it would suffice to control that center, on the inside of the figure; the limbs, which are really nothing but pendulums, follow of themselves, in a mechanical way, without further aid. . . ."
>
> I replied that I had always thought this activity something quite mindless, rather like turning the crank on a hand organ.

"By no means," he answered. "On the contrary, the relation of his finger movements to the movements of the puppets attached to them is something quite precise. . . ."

In his foreword to *The Final Fate of the Alligators,* Edward Hoagland observes that stuttering, as a disability, is almost certain to affect a writer and his work. And he alludes to Edmund Wilson's famous essay, "The Wound and the Bow," on *Philoctetes,* the great and penultimate play of Sophocles. In that play, we find conjoined in the hero an invincible power with a seemingly incurable wound; and the question arises, through the play's action, as to whether the tie between the two is inseparable—whether the power or gift will remain if the wound is healed. First through compassion, then the physician's art, the wound *is* healed, in the play's resolution, and the gift retained.

Perhaps some stutterers think of themselves as having been compensated for their disability by some special power; but most regard it as a cross. The artists among them are probably different in that respect, insofar as their inability to communicate in the normal way acts as a spur to creative expression. But I doubt that many, if they could awake one morning to a tongue untangled, would not count it the Day of Jubilee.

There was a good deal of surprise some years back when the testing of college stutterers indicated that they were more intelligent on average than their peers. Subsequently it was realized that it required extra aptitude for anyone with a developmental disorder to make it to college in the first place. Wider testing found that stutterers on the whole were neither more nor less intelligent than anybody else.

All human defects are ambiguous, and from time immemorial those with apparent deformities have been treated in contradictory ways. The same unfeeling ancient Romans who caged speech defectives like animals and mocked them along the Appian Way, revered Vergil as their greatest poet; and Saint Thomas à Becket (likewise afflicted) was exalted to the pinnacle of the Church in England by a people who seared the lips of the stuttering "possessed." Aristotle and Hippocrates thought stuttering a sign of worth, and Henri Le Strange in his sympathetic biography of King Charles I (published in 1654) tells us that the king's impediment was "to wise men an index of his wisdom . . . since there was never, or very rarely, known a fool that stammered." Bacon, Carlyle, and others have echoed the same theme, which forms a gratifying (if skewed) historical counterweight to the more typical social ridicule. More balanced was the view expressed by Sir Richard Steele in *The Tatler* in 1710: "A man that stammers, if he has Understanding, is to be attended with Patience." I think most stutterers would be satisfied with that.

Although the U.S. Immigration and Naturalization Service at one time reportedly barred stutterers as mental defectives from entry into the United States, today under Public Law 94-142, stuttering is appropriately recognized as a physical handicap and public schools are obliged to provide assistance to any afflicted child.

In our end is our beginning. If we return to the biblical story of Moses, the most ancient of all known stutterers, we will find it there implied that stuttering is inborn. "Who hath made man's mouth?" exclaims Yahweh (Exodus 4:11), in one of his testy rebukes to Moses "or who maketh the dumb, or deaf, or the seeing or the blind?" Later rabbinical tradition, contemplating the prophet's life, allowed stuttering a physical cause. "When Moses was still an infant," according to one time-honored tale, "the Pharaoh became suspicious that he was no ordinary child and eventually might try to usurp his throne." So he arranged a superstitious test. He placed the infant between two platters, one strewn with glowing coals, the other heaped with jewels. Should Moses choose the latter (representing the riches of the kingdom), he was to die. Moses reached at once with delight for the jewels, but "at the last instant an angel diverted his arm" and caused him to put the searing coals instead into his mouth. From that moment on, he stuttered; but he lived, and he grew to eminence, and delivered his people out of bondage to the borders of the Promised Land. Whatever other lessons may be drawn from this curious tale, perhaps it may also be surmised from the angel's intercession that even stuttering in life's labyrinthine journey can sometimes prove a blessing in disguise.

# Notes

For abbreviations used in the notes, and for full titles and other bibliographical information on books, articles, interviews, and other documents cited, the reader is referred to the Bibliography.

*Part One: Anatomy of Melancholy*
Chapter 1
    17  *"You know there is a way out":* C. Woodruff Starkweather, quoted in Ecenbarger, "Speaking the Truth About Stuttering," p. 52.
    18  *"the most complex disorganization":* Bluemel, "Concepts of Stammering," p. 30.
    18  *"The girl imprisoned":* Auden and Isherwood, *The Ascent of F6,* p. 41.

18 "Feminas verba balba decent": Horace, Ep. 2, 1.33.

18 *"Some may imagine"*: J. Hunt, *Stammering and Stuttering*, p. 4.

19 *"Courage: your tongue has left"*: Dugan, *Poems*, "Stutterer," p. 55.

20 *"I give my stuttering to you"*: Van Riper, "Historical Approaches to Stuttering," p. 39.

Chapter 2

22 *"soonest"*: Burton, *Anatomy of Melancholy*, p. 99.

22 *"anguish of mind"*: Ibid., p. 149.

23 *"a certain reserve"*: Quoted in Froeschels, "Survey of the Early Literature on Stuttering," p. 89.

23 *"Stammering [in a child] rises as"*: Dickens, "Psellism—The Act of Stammering," *Household Words*, p. 14.

23 *"the conversation of the soul"*: O'Neill, *Speech and Speech Disorders*, p. 34.

23 *"the stream of thought"*: Plato, *Collected Dialogues*, p. 1009.

24 *"not just a physical function."*: O'Neill, *Speech and Speech Disorders*, p. 202.

24 *"In a village"*: Bede, *The Ecclesiastical History of the English People*, p. 268.

26 *"most satisfactory appellation"*: O'Neill, *Speech and Speech Disorders*, p. 3.

26 *"one who utters"*: Quoted in *ibid.*, p. 100.

28 *"vibrations that occur"*: Webster, *The Precision Fluency Shaping Program*, vol. 2, p. 35.

29 *"the sentential system"*: Curlee and Perkins, eds., *Nature and Treatment of Stuttering*, p. 262.

29 *"That's a lot"*: R. L. Webster, quoted in *Family Circle Magazine*, "The Ordeal of Annie Glenn," p. 1.

30 *"pile up like"*: Van Riper, *Speech Correction*, p. 26.

31 *"snort like a rhinoceros"*: Hoagland, *Heart's Desire*, p. 131.

31 *"I see the repulsive symptoms"*: Updike, *Self-Consciousness: Memoirs*, p. 80.

31 *"a paroxysm of stuttering"*: Quoted in Rieber, ed., *The Problem of Stuttering*, p. 163.

31 *"when in truth"*: Updike, *Self-Consciousness: Memoirs*, p. 88.

32 *"The human body"*: Greene and Wells, *The Cause and Cure of Speech Disorders*, pp. 64–65.

33 *"My first morning"*: Quoted in Schwartz, *Stop Stuttering*, p. 105.

33 *"jump up and down"*: Starkweather, Gottwald, and Halfond, *Stuttering Prevention*, p. 10.

33 *"squeeze the words out"*: *Ibid.*, p. 10.

33 *"who could release"*: Schwartz, *Stuttering Solved*, p. 17.

34 *"the whole house"*: Murray, *A Stutterer's Story*, p. 117.

34 *"[My stammer] has assumed"*: Quoted in *Letting Go*, no. 8-9, August–September 1992.

36 *"Think of yourself"*: Patrusky, "The Secret Ben Can't Keep," p. 15.

36 *"there was no obvious"*: Quoted in Motion, *Philip Larkin*, p. 9.

37 *"elaborate, stilted, pedantic"*: Sheehan, ed., *Stuttering: Research and Therapy*, p. 28.

37 *"Here's the fare"*: Quoted in D. Miller, "St-st-stuttering: It Isn't Hopeless," p. 72.

37 *"I could never say anything"*: Kazin, *A Walker in the City*, pp. 22–23.

38 *"bleach out"*: Hoagland, Interviews with author, August 17, 1993.

38 *"are able to pose"*: Van Riper, *Speech Correction*, p. 26.

39 *"a striking instance"*: Melville, *Billy Budd*, pp. 17–18.

39 *"hardly speak"*: Creighton, *Margaret Drabble*, p. 21.

39 *"the axe was always"*: Quoted in *ibid.*, p. 22.

39 *"often accused me"*: Jones, *Voices and Silences*, p. 41.

40 *"[Kim was] a most attentive"*: E. Philby, *Kim Philby*, p. 52.

41 *"The trial was held"*: Knightley, *Philby*, p. 200.

42 *"Any mechanism"*: Updike, *Self-Consciousness: Memoirs*, p. 87.

42 *"an attempt to avoid"*: Ecenbarger, "When Words Fail," p. 14.

42 *"hand over little slips"*: Quoted in Compton, *Stammering*, p. 45.

43 *"This stammer in my address"*: Goldsmith, *She Stoops to Conquer*, Act 2, Scene 1.

43 *"I was a depressed"*: Boberg, "The Winding Trails of Therapy," p. 4.

43 *"while I was allowed"*: Quoted in Schwartz, *Stuttering Solved*, p. 41.

43 *"couldn't collect"*: Ecenbarger, *When Words Fail*, p. 14.

44 *"were taught to paint"* and

45 *"enthusiastic and full"*: Murray, *A Stutterer's Story*, p. 100.

45 *"sitting around with a bib"*: Congressman Frank Wolf, in *Letting Go*, vol. 14, No. 2, p. 4.

*Part Two: Conundrum*
Chapter 3

49 *"to speak haltingly"*: Quoted in Eldridge, *A History of the Treatment of Speech Disorders*, p. 3.

49 *"O God! Cut through"*: Quoted in Van Riper, *Speech Correction*, p. 306.

50 "ischnophonos kai traulos": Herodotus, *History*, p. 294.

50 *"the omission of one particular"*: Quoted in O'Neill, *Speech and Speech Disorders*, p. 40.

50 *"hesitancy"*: Quoted in O'Neill, *Speech and Speech Disorders*, p. 40.

50 *"Why is it that"*: Ibid., p. 40.

51 *"into position for uttering"*: Quoted in Eldridge, *A History of the Treatment*, p. 15.

51 *"thinking of fresh things"*: Quoted in Rieber and Wollock, "The Historical Roots," p. 10.

52 *"to immerse his head"*: Quoted in ibid., p. 60.

52 *"tongue-tied from birth"*: Rieber and Wollock, "The Historical Roots," p. 134.

52 *"undercut so far"*: Quoted in Eldridge, *A History of the Treatment,* p. 20. See also Rieber and Wollock, "The Historical Roots," p. 135.

52 *"midwives used to cut away"*: Quoted in Rieber and Wollock, "The Historical Roots," p. 135.

53 *"that human beings were a microcosm"*: O'Neill, *Speech and Speech Disorders,* p. 108.

54 *"the actual disease"*: Wollock, "Communication Disorders," p. 17.

54 *"unless one or more"*: O'Neill, *Speech and Speech Disorders,* p. 109.

55 *"that the membrane itself"*: Quoted in Rieber and Wollock, "The Historical Roots," p. 136.

55 *"there is a period"*: Quoted in O'Neill, *Speech and Speech Disorders,* p. 108.

56 *"deep thought, immoderate Venus"*: Quoted in Rieber and Wollock, "The Historical Roots," p. 131.

56 *"since before that time"*: Quoted in *ibid.,* p. 140.

56 *"That these may be"*: Quoted in *ibid.,* p. 140.

58 *"Whan Stuttynge"*: Boorde, *A Breviary of Healthe,* p. xli.

58 *"I pr'ythee, tell me"*: Shakespeare, *As You Like It,* Act 3, Scene 2.

59 *"singular good remedie"*: Quoted in Wollock, "Communication Disorders in Renaissance Italy," p. 117.

59 *"Divers, we see, doe Stut"*: Bacon, *Sylva Sylvarum,* Cent. IV, Sec. 386.

60 *"It is a worlde"*: Palsgrave, *Fullonius' Comedye of Acolastus,* Act 3, Sc., 1.44.

60 *"Hee lookes bigge"*: Jonson, *The Poetaster,* Act 5, Scene 5.

60 *"If it [stuttering] do come"*: Boorde, *A Breviary of Healthe,* p. xlii.

61 *"the contraction"*: Quoted in J. Hunt, *Stammering and Stuttering,* p. 66.

61 *"I do not believe"*: Maugham, *Selected Works,* p. 99.

62　*"Fortune did never favour one"*: Herrick, "Fortunes favours."

62　*"of all other men most,"* etc.: Lenaghan, ed., *Caxton's Aesop,* p. 1.

63　*"Lord, open my breast"*: Arberry, trans., Koran, p. 340.

66　*"From that moment on"*: Encyclopaedia Britannica, vol. 4, p. 9.

67　*"his name was synonymous"*: Ibid., p. 9.

68　*"unfinished by nature"*: Quoted in Scramuzza, *The Emperor Claudius,* p. 35.

68　*"incapable of acting"*: Quoted in *ibid.,* p. 36.

68　*"slobbered horribly"*: Suetonius, *The Twelve Caesars,* p. 199.

68　*"in important matters"*: Quoted in Scramuzza, *The Emperor Claudius,* p. 38.

68　*"unclear"*: Ibid., p. 37.

69　*"obstinate mutual enmity"*: Encyclopaedia Britannica, vol. 3, p. 360.

69　*"His health"*: Suetonius, *The Twelve Caesars,* p. 200.

69　*"came to see the boy"*: Quoted in Gregg, *King Charles I,* p. 10.

70　*"very wilful and obstinate"*: Quoted in *ibid.,* p. 12.

70　*"nothing undignified"*: Quoted in Hibbert, *Charles I,* p. 30.

71　*"Because I am unfit"*: Quoted in D'Israeli, *Commentaries on the Life and Reign,* p. 21.

71　*"he had a quicker"*: Quoted in Bowle, *Charles I,* p. 7.

71　*"gave audience easily"*: Quoted in Bowle, *Charles I,* p. 6.

71　*"very majestic and steady"*: Quoted in Carleton, *Charles I,* p. 355.

71　*"he stammered nothing at all"*: Quoted in Bowle, *Charles I,* p. 7.

71　*"a just judgment,"* etc.: Quoted in Maddison, *The Life of the Honourable Robert Boyle,* p. 4.

72　*"to fix his volatile fancy"*: Thompson, *Robert Boyle,* p. 10.

72　*"he proceeded without"*: Quoted in Maddison, *The Life of the Honourable Robert Boyle,* p. 188.

73  *"'Tis almost amazing"*: Thomas Prince, quoted in Mather, *Selections*, xxv–xxvi.

73  *"an Odd, Starv'd, Lank"*: Mather, *Manuductio ad Ministerium*, p. 30.

74  *"I know of one who"*: Mather, *The Angel of Bethesda*, p. 231.

74  *"Inhumane Derision"*: *Ibid.*, p. 236.

74  *"a Thing as much despaired of"*: *Ibid.*, p. 231.

74  *"to oblige himself"*: Mather, *Diary*, vol. 1, p. 2, n. 2.

74  *"drawling . . . little short"*: Mather, *The Angel of Bethesda*, p. 231.

74  *"By this Deliberation"*: Quoted in *ibid.*, p. 231.

74  *"to threaten . . . to render me"*: Quoted in Silverman, *The Life and Times of Cotton Mather*, p. 19.

75  *"The Original of this Infirmity"*: Mather, *The Angel of Bethesda*, p. 230.

Chapter 4

76  *"some of those persons"*: Quoted in MacNamee, "Normativity in 18th Century Discourse," p. 417.

77  *"the melody dictates to them"*: *Ibid.*

78  *"a companionable, brilliant soul"*: Quoted in Kupferberg, *The Mendelssohns*, p. 11.

78  *"a collision between many ideas"*: Eldridge, *A History of the Treatment*, p. 36.

78  *"Great you call Demosthenes"*: Quoted in *ibid.*, p. 15.

79  *"the chief intellectual"*: King-Hele, *Doctor of Revolution*, p. 2.

80  *"and all that sustains it"*: *Ibid.*, p. 18.

80  *"stammered extremely"*: Seward, *Memoirs of the Life of Dr. Darwin*, p. 2.

80  *"the closest attention"*: Seward, quoted in King-Hele, *Doctor of Revolution*, p. 188.

80  *"always revenged it"*: Seward, *Memoirs of the Life of Dr. Darwin*, p. 2.

81 *"Wine, women, warmth"*: Quoted in King-Hele, *Doctor of Revolution*, p. 51.

81 *"to the pleasure of the first"*: Quoted in Krause, *Erasmus Darwin*, p. 167.

81 *"when any object of vision"*: Darwin, *Zoonomia*, vol. 1, pp. 146–47.

81 *"eating an almost immeasurable"*: King-Hele, *Doctor of Revolution*, p. 187.

82 *"high state of vinous,"* etc.: Quoted in King-Hele, *Doctor of Revolution*, p. 51.

82 *"corresponding fear of failure,"* etc.: Quoted in Rieber and Wollock, "The Historical Roots," p. 11.

82 *"become dissevered"*: Darwin, *Zoonomia*, vol. 1, p. 107.

82 *"The art of curing"*: Quoted in Rieber and Wollock, "The Historical Roots," p. 11.

83 *"clear contoured sounds"*: Quoted in *ibid.*, p. 88.

83 *"by the streams of air"*: Quoted in *ibid.*, p. 88.

83 *"much like a human voice,"* etc.: *Ibid.*

84 *"a local yokel"*: Quoted in *ibid.*

84 *"You will be a disgrace"*: Darwin, *The Autobiography*, p. 28.

Chapter 5

85 *"caused by a general debility"*: Eldridge, *A History of the Treatment*, p. 38.

85 *"confused and indistinct"*: Quoted in J. Hunt, *Stammering and Stuttering*, p. 73.

86 *"nervous affection"*: Quoted in *ibid.*, p. 74.

86 *"You must shake"*: Quoted in *ibid.*, p. 75.

86 *"the cerebral irradiation"*: Quoted in *ibid.*, p. 76.

86 *"the cause of stuttering consists"*: Quoted in *ibid.*, pp. 82–83.

87 *"discovery hitherto made by none."*: Quoted in J. Hunt, *Stammering and Stuttering*, p. 79.

87 *"speaking in a subdued"*: Quoted in *ibid.*, p. 94.

87 *"be joined together"*: Quoted in *ibid.*, p. 89.

88 *"trying to speak"*: Quoted in Compton, *Stammering*, p. 133.

88 *"to run smoothly"*: Quoted in *ibid.*, p. 136.

88 *"not larger than"*: Quoted in Rieber, ed., *The Problem of Stuttering*, p. 146.

88 *"But passion"*: Quoted in *ibid.*, pp. 146–47.

89 *"a* conflict *between"*: Quoted in Rieber, ed. *The Problem of Stuttering*, p. 149.

89 *"Wherever two or more"*: Quoted in *ibid.*, p. 147.

89 *"without choking himself"*: Quoted in *ibid.*, p. 151.

89 *"In January, 1833"*: J. Hunt, *Stammering and Stuttering*, p. 45.

90 *"Stammering originates"*: Quoted in Rieber, ed., *The Problem of Stuttering*, p. 160.

90 *"I may allude"*: Quoted in J. Hunt, *Stammering and Stuttering*, pp. 160–62.

91 *"the sound is continued"*: Quoted in *ibid.*, p. 168.

91 *"to be spoken"*: Quoted in Jonas, *Stuttering: The Disorder of Many Theories*, p. 19.

92 *"while biting down"*: Quoted in *ibid.*, p. 19.

93 *"because there the Organs"*: Quoted in MacNamee, "Normativity," p. 417.

93 *"Her felow did stammer and stut"*: Skelton, "The Tunnynge of Elyonour Rummyng," line 339.

93 *"A Man . . . [doth] Stammer, Stut"*: Holme, *The Academie of Armoury*, p. 389.

94 *"a defective articulation of certain sounds"*: J. Hunt, *Stammering and Stuttering*, p. 115.

94 *"The idea lately suggested itself"*: Quoted in Burdin, "The Surgical Treatment of Stammering," pp. 44–45.

94 *"highly intelligent and talented"*: Quoted in Stevenson, *The Surgery of Stammering*, p. 534.

95 *"The patient was seated"*: Quoted in Burdin, "The Surgical Treatment," pp. 45–46.

96  *"There is some blood"*: Quoted in Stevenson, "The Surgery of Stammering," p. 540.

96  *"immediately beset with sufferers"*: Ibid., p. 47.

97  *"the free elevation of the tip"*: Quoted in ibid., p. 60.

97  *"taken by surprise"*: Quoted in ibid., p. 53.

98  *"stammered out that they"*: Quoted in ibid., p. 543.

98  *"Within the last few months"*: Quoted in Burdin, "The Surgical Treatment," p. 55.

98  *"We shall have conical and oblique"*: Quoted in ibid., p. 50.

100  *"who had a very asymmetrical skull"*: Quoted in Lebrun and Hoops, eds., *Neurolinguistic Approaches to Stuttering*, p. 86.

100  *"into the cancelled structure"*: Quoted in Burdin, "The Surgical Treatment," p. 61.

101  *"distended like a sail"*: Quoted in ibid., pp. 61–62.

101  *"have a parental or collateral relation"*: J. Hunt, *Stammering and Stuttering*, p. 41.

102  *"to speak consciously"*: Ibid., p. 137.

102  *"mental tranquillity and self-control."*: Ibid., p. 141.

102  *"defrauded"*: Quoted in Barnett, *Charles Lamb*, p. 24.

103  *"magnificent"*: Quoted in ibid., p. 28.

103  *"grunted once or twice"*: Courtney, *Young Charles Lamb*, p. 348.

103  *"All full up inside?"*: Quoted in Ecenbarger, "When Words Fail," p. 11.

103  *"a solvent of speech."*: Quoted in Barnett, *Charles Lamb*, p. 34.

103  *"the ligaments which"*: Quoted in Barnett, *Charles Lamb*, p. 34.

104  *"I hesitated in my speech"*: Quoted in Courtney, *Young Charles Lamb*, p. 99.

104  *"a vague sense"*: Quoted in Courtney, *Young Charles Lamb*, p. 49.

104  *"I did nothing for"*: Quoted in Thompson, *Leigh Hunt*, p. 15.

105  *"almost every disorder"*: Blainey, *Immortal Boy*, p. 5.

105 *"his morbid fear"*: B. Miller, *Leigh Hunt's Relations*, p. 6.

105 *"an ultra-tender"*: Quoted in Blainey, *Immortal Boy*.

105 *"sighed compulsively"*: Ibid., p. 116.

105 *"The worse my stammering"*: Quoted in *ibid.*, p. 11.

106 *"nerves ruined by croup"*: Thorp, *Charles Kingsley*, p. 10.

106 *"manly"*: Quoted in Compton, *Stammering*, p. 143.

106 *"the Cave, on account"*: Quoted in Collins, *Charles Kingsley*, p. 45.

107 *"I could be as great"*: Quoted in Thorp, *Charles Kingsley*, p. 165.

107 *"Learn well your grammer"*: Quoted in Newark, *Not Good at Talking*, p. 60.

108 *"By this means"*: Clark, *Lewis Carroll*, p. 118.

108 *"Looking straight in front"*: Quoted in *ibid.*, p. 118.

108 *"A sermon would be quite"*: Quoted in *ibid.*, p. 120.

109 *"Read service in the afternoon."*: Quoted in *ibid.*, p. 186.

109 *"Read the first verse"*: Quoted in *ibid.*, p. 258.

109 *"We used to sit"*: Quoted in *Encyclopaedia Britannica*, vol. 2, p. 902.

110 *"I think all you say"*: Quoted in Gattegno, *Lewis Carroll*, p. 65.

110 *"a nightmare of constant,"* etc.: Wallace, *The Agony of Lewis Carroll*, p. 13.

110 *"the destructive world"*: Ibid., p. 211.

111 *"And so wider but we"*: Joyce, *Finnegan's Wake*, p. 115.

112 *"toy with statistical permutations"*: Lebrun and Hoops, eds., *Neurolinguistic Approaches to Stuttering*, p. 126.

112 *"He confirms an observation"*: Quoted in Murray, *A Stutterer's Story*, p. 100.

112 *"collapsed into silence"*: Kaplan, *Henry James*, p. 58.

113 *"the great Victorian houses"*: Encyclopaedia Britannica, vol. 6, p. 486.

113 *"his manner"*: Quoted in Markow-Totevy, *Henry James*, p. 14.

113  *"Henry James could not say":* Quoted in Pirie, *Henry James,* p. 28.

113  *"hesitant 'm-m's":* Quoted in *ibid.,* p. 31.

113  *"the anguished facial contortions":* Quoted in *ibid.,* p. 128.

113  *"almost invariably broke up":* Quoted in *ibid.,* p. 75.

113  *"The scene was":* Quoted in *ibid.*

114  *"was largely composed":* Quoted in Nowell-Smith, *The Legend of the Master,* p. 14.

114  *"the most popular":* Quoted in Pirie, *Henry James,* p. 76.

114  *"we went and had tea":* Quoted in *ibid.,* p. 133.

115  *"In conversation he was":* Quoted in Nowell-Smith, *The Legend of the Master,* p. 11.

115  *"The greatest compliment":* Quoted in *ibid.,* p. 11.

115  *"he talked as if":* Quoted in *ibid.*

116  *"His slow way of speech":* Quoted in *ibid.,* p. 13.

116  *"I had never heard":* Quoted in Pirie, *Henry James,* p. 140.

117  *"exactly like":* Quoted in Kaplan, *Henry James,* p. 465.

117  *"its amplifications, hesitations":* Quoted in *ibid.,* p. 128.

117  *"Nothing would be further":* Quoted in *ibid.,* p. 111.

118  *"She will never assert herself":* Quoted in W. E. Barton, *The Life of Clara Barton,* p. 21.


Chapter 6

121  *"failure of confidence":* Bloodstein, *Stuttering,* p. 13.

121  *"If we examine":* Quoted in Van Riper, "Historical Approaches," p. 43.

122  *"The boy who has no great fear":* Quoted in Boome and Richardson, *The Nature and Treatment of Stuttering,* p. 14.

122  *"the vocal and buccal":* Lebrun and Hoops, eds., *Neurolinguistic Approaches to Stuttering,* p. 29.

122  *"the act of giving out":* Ibid., p. 29.

122  *"persistence into adult life":* Coriat, "The Psychoanalytic Conception of Stuttering," p. 167.

123  *"In the pregenital stage": Ibid.,* p. 168.

123  *"Stammerers will often bite": Ibid.,* p. 169.

123  *"a protective mechanism":* Coriat, "Stammering—A Psychoanalytic Interpretation," p. 5.

124  *"primal sexual pleasure,"* etc.: *Ibid.,* p. 10.

124  *"peculiar hand movements,"* etc.: *Ibid.,* p. 7.

124  *"no matter how frequently": Ibid.,* p. 15.

124  *"a latent homosexual":* Coriat, "Stammering—A Psychoanalytic Interpretation," p. 45.

124  *"The tongue has become a displaced"* etc.: Coriat, "The Psychoanalytic Conception," p. 170.

125  *"their whole attitude":* Quoting a colleague of like mind in Coriat, "Stammering—A Psychoanalytic Interpretation," p. 50.

125  *"are always hopeful,"* etc.: *Ibid.,* pp. 50–51.

126  *"the dominant hemisphere determined":* Bloodstein, *Stuttering,* p. 30.

126  *"Needle electrodes were inserted":* Quoted in Murray, *A Stutterer's Story,* p. 88.

127  *"simultaneous talking and writing":* Quoted in Sheehan, "Current Issues in Stuttering and Recovery," p. 294.

127  *"an inherited predisposition":* Webster, "Establishment of Fluent Speech in Stutterers," p. 4.

128  *"inherit peculiar neuropathic":* Boome and Richardson, *The Nature and Treatment of Stuttering,* p. 16.

128  *"A few days after I arrived":* Johnson, *Stuttering and What You Can Do About It,* p. 25.

129  *"ten years and countless bruises":* Quoted in Jonas, *Stuttering: The Disorder of Many Theories,* p. 29.

129  *"[It] came to me":* Quoted in Ahlbach, *To Say What Is Ours,* vol. 7, p. 31.

130  *"that would be tolerable":* Quoted in *ibid.*

131  *"Stuttering is not something":* Quoted in Murray, *A Stutterer's Story,* p. 88.

132 *"stuttering begins not"*: Johnson, *Stuttering in Children and Adults*, p. 18.

132 *"nothing is more adapted"*: Guttmann, *Gymnastics of the Voice*, p. 237.

133 *"by drawing attention to the mechanism"*: Boome and Richardson, *The Nature and Treatment of Stuttering*, pp. 11, 81.

133 *"The female has more control"*: Quoted in Boberg and Kully, "A Retrospective Look at Stuttering Therapy," p. 2.

133 *"All travelers"*: Hunt, *Stammering and Stuttering*, p. 94.

134 *"their freedom from mental anxieties"*: J. Hunt, *Stammering and Stuttering*, p. 39.

135 *"Stuttering is a disorder of the social"*: Sheehan, ed., *Stuttering: Research and Therapy*, p. 4.

135 *"to become a stutterer all the way"*: Ibid., p. 8.

135 *"The experience of speaking normally"*: Ibid., p. 7.

136 *"It happens when I feel"*: Updike, *Self-Consciousness: Memoirs*, p. 80.

136 *"You stutter, I think"*: New York Observer, March 15, 1993.

136 *"I did not, at heart"*: Updike, *Self-Consciousness: Memoirs*, p. 80.

136 *"I tried to read:"* Ibid., p. 80.

136 *"in the wrong"*: Ibid., p. 85.

137 *"a bored"*: Ibid., p. 80

137 *"if a stutterer were to forget"*: Bloodstein, in Curlee and Perkins, eds., *Nature and Treatment of Stuttering*, p. 174.

137 *"Almost anyone would be able"*: Bloodstein, *Stuttering*, p. 9.

137 *"Confused and embarrassed"*: Barbara, *The Psychodynamics of Stuttering*, p. 65.

138 *"He may feel"*: Ibid., pp. 111–12.

138 *"neurotic tendencies"* and *"personality peculiarities"*: Bender, *The Personality Structure of Stuttering*, p. 125.

139 *"it is remarkable"*: Brady, "The Pharmacology of Stuttering," p. 1310.

139 *"claustrophobia, isolating fear"*: Hoagland, *The Final Fate of the Alligators*, p. 15.

139 *"I began to write novels"*: Quoted in Hepburn, *The Mind and Heart of Arnold Bennett*, pp. xvi–xvii.

140 *"I think there was some obscure"*: Quoted in Allen, *Arnold Bennett*, p. 19.

140 *"You can't have a baby"*: Quoted in *ibid.*, p. 32.

140 *"it was painful to watch"*: S. Maugham, Preface to *The Old Wives' Tale*, p. x.

140 *"beating his knee"*: Morgan, *Maugham*, p. 350.

141 *"the hesitancy of his speech"*: Drabble, *Arnold Bennett*, p. 73.

141 *"made his prose pithy"*: R. Maugham, *Conversations with Willie*, p. 122.

141 *"I have no doubt"*: Quoted in Naik, *W. Somerset Maugham*, p. 22.

141 *"I think many people"*: Quoted in *ibid.*, p. 23.

142 *"Sit down, you fool!"*: Quoted in Calder, *Willie*, p. 13.

142 *"suddenly two men"*: Quoted in R. Maugham, *Conversations with Willie*, p. 121.

143 *"Well, every novelist"*: Quoted in *ibid.*, p. 283.

144 *"until he came to a passage"*: Quoted in Morgan, *Maugham*, p. 557.

144 *"self-inflicted. The stammerer"*: *Ibid.*, p. 16.

145 *"a clubfoot is something"*: *Ibid.*, p. 16.

145 *"the sudden demand"*: Calder, *Willie*, p. 11.

145 *"would frequently complain"*: Calder, *W. Somerset Maugham and the Quest for Freedom*, p. 7.

145 *"Psychologically, the stammerer"*: *Ibid.*, p. 56.

145 *"He can speak in"*: *Ibid.*, pp. 56–57.

146 *"stammered over commonplace"*: Quoted in Calder, *Willie*, p. 11.

146 *"He entered my consulting room"*: Quoted in Compton, *Stammering*, p. 97.

146  *"I have been seeing Logue"*: Quoted in Newark, *Not Good at Talking*, p. 19.

147  *"I'm quite unprepared for it"*: Quoted in *ibid.*, p. 21.

147  *"no monarch ever succeeded"*: Ibid., p. 21.

147  *"always an ordeal"*: Quoted in *ibid.*, p. 21.

147  *"I got the BBC"*: Murray, *A Stutterer's Story*, p. 48.

148  *"The Spanish ships"*: R. S. Churchill, *Winston S. Churchill: Youth*, p. 252.

148  *"about 5' 8" tall"*: Quoted in *ibid.*, p. 481.

149  *"painful and embarrassing"*:  Birkenhead,  *Churchill, 1874–1922*, p. 113.

149  *"I wrote out"*: Fisher, *My Darling Clementine*, p. 25.

150  *"For anyone with a stutter"*: Quoted in Brome, *Aneurin Bevan*, p. 31.

150  *"You stammer in speech"*: Quoted in Krug, *Aneurin Bevan*, p. 35.

150  *"It might be a word"*: Brome, *Aneurin Bevan*, p. 10.

150  *"he not so much mastered"*: Ibid., p. 3.

151  *"my officers discovered"*: Shute, *Slide Rule*, p. 26.

151  *"I was stammering"*: Ibid.

151  *"could hardly have invaded"*: Ibid., p. 29.

152  *"caused her agony"*: Glendinning, *Elizabeth Bowen*, p. 26.

152  *"it became very much part"*: Ibid., p. 27.

153  *"lovely whistling stammer"*: Quoted in Craig, *Elizabeth Bowen*, p. 121.

153  *"the stammering flow"*: Quoted in Glendinning, *Elizabeth Bowen*, p. 170.

153  *"completely disappeared"*: Ibid., p. 300.

153  *"vocal handcuffs"*: Hoagland, *Heart's Desire*, p. 132.

153  *"the closest thing to speech"*: Hoagland, Interview with author, August 17, 1993.

153  *"more unsettling to other people"*: Ibid., p. 131.

153  *"that it didn't seem"*: Ibid.

154  *"to take command"*: Ibid.

154 *"probably the symptom"*: Carleton, *Charles I*, p. 59.

154 *"Heredity, pre-natal disturbance"*: Gregg, *King Charles I*, p. 13.

154 *"over-rigorous pot-training"*: Drabble, *Arnold Bennett*, p. 33.

## Part Three: Deliverance
Chapter 7

159 *"The aim should be"*: Quoted in Gregory, *Controversies About Stuttering Therapy*, p. 76.

163 *"the vildest stumbling stutterer"*: Marston, *The Scourge of Villanie* (1598), ix, 1.5.

164 *"with the same impulse"*: Quoted in Miller, "St-st-stuttering: It Isn't Hopeless," p. 73.

164 *"Never again"*: Quoted in *ibid.*, p. 73.

164 *"By the time I was 40"*: Rappoport, "Clinic Helps Actor Alleviate Stutter," p. 1.

165 *"One day in or around 1950"*: Bloodstein, *Stuttering*, p. 92.

168 *"probably no more than"*: Van Riper, *Speech Correction*, p. 317.

169 *"a need for the stutterer"*: Wall and Myers, *Clinical Management of Childhood Stuttering*, p. 28.

171 *"possibly derived"*: Brady, "The Pharmacology of Stuttering," p. 1310.

172 *"overshooting"*: Webster, "Establishment of Fluent Speech in Stutterers," p. 7.

172 *"loci of effects"*: *Ibid.*, p. 6.

172 *"a motor control disorder"*: *Ibid.*, p. 1.

173 *"a series of tiny"*: Webster, "Precision Fluency Shaping Program Prospectus," 1974.

173 *"For a stutterer to speak fluently"*: Webster, *The Precision Fluency Shaping Program*, vol. 2, p. 11.

174 *"at the level of muscle activity."*: Webster, *The Precision Fluency Shaping Program*, vol. 2, p. 124.

175 *"You know if it's right"*: Catherine Otto, Interview with author, December 16, 1993.

175 *"Stuttering is not something"*: Quoted in Murray, *A Stutterer's Story*, p. 88.

175 *"When you entered this program"*: Webster, *The Precision Fluency Shaping Program*, vol. 2, p. 86.

178 *"If we vibrate the skull"*: Webster, Interview with author, March 24, 1993.

180 *"because of a maturational delay"*: Boberg and Webster, "Stuttering: Current Status of Theory and Therapy," p. 1158.

180 *"Methods that teach stutterers"*: Bloodstein, *Stuttering*, p. 161.

181 *"Why did fluency controls"*: *Letting Go*, vol. 8, No. 6, p. 6.

182 *"At some point, like the Zen archer"*: *Ibid.*, vol. 13, No. 11, Autumn supplement, p. 2.

183 *". . . until the frog in fun"*: Murray, *A Stutterer's Story*, p. 158.

183 *" 'Each movement,' he said,"*: Quoted in P. Miller, ed., *An Abyss Deep Enough*, pp. 211–12.

185 *"to wise men an index"*: Quoted in D'Israeli, *Commentaries on the Life and Reign of Charles the First*, vol. 1, p. 21.

185 *"A man that stammers"*: Steele, *The Tatler*, No. 244, p. 2.

186 *"When Moses was still an infant"*: G. M. Siegel, "Moses the Stutterer," in *Letting Go*, vol. 7, No. 1, p. 9.

# Bibliography

Abbreviations

*AJP American Journal of Psychiatry*

*AMJ American Medical Journal*

*ASHA American Speech Language Hearing Association*

*BHM Bulletin of the History of Medicine*

*JAP Journal of Abnormal Psychology*

*JASP Journal of Abnormal and Social Psychology*

*JCD Journal of Communication Disorders*

*JFD Journal of Fluency Disorders*

*JNMD Journal of Nervous and Mental Disorders*

*JSD Journal of Speech Disorders*

*JSHD Journal of Speech and Hearing Disorders*

*JSHR Journal of Speech and Hearing Research*

*NC Nervous Child*

Adams, M. "A Clinical Strategy for Differentiating the Normally Nonfluent Child and the Incipient Stutterer," *JFD,* 2 (1977), 141–48.

Ahlbach, J. (Ed.) *To Say What Is Ours: The Ten Best Years of "Letting Go."* National Stuttering Project. San Francisco, 1990.

Ainger, A. *Charles Lamb.* London, 1988.

Allen, W. *Arnold Bennett.* Denver, 1949.

Appelt, A. *Stammering and Its Permanent Cure.* London, 1911.

Anderson, L. O. "Stuttering and Allied Disorders," *Comparative Psychology Monographs,* 1 (No. 4, March 1923), 1–75. Baltimore, 1923.

Andrews, G., and M. Harris. (Eds.) *The Syndrome of Stuttering.* London, 1964.

Andrews, G., A. Craig, A. Feyer, S. Hoddinott, P. Howie, and M. Neilson. "Stuttering: A Review of Research Findings and Theories Circa 1982," *JFD,* 48 (1983), 226–46.

Andrews, G., and M. Dozsa. "Haloperidol and the Treatment of Stuttering," *JFD,* 2 (1977), 217–24.

Andrews, G., and R. J. Ingham. "An Approach to the Evaluation of Stuttering Therapy," *JSHD,* 15 (1972), 296–302.

Andrews, G., P. Quinn, and W. Sorby. "Stuttering: An Investigation into Cerebral Dominance for Speech," *Journal of Neurology, Neurosurgery and Psychiatry,* 35 (1972), 414–18.

Arberry, A. J. (Trans.) Koran. London, 1955.

Arch, M. E. "Now I Can Talk," *Hollins Communications Research Institute.* Roanoke, VA, January 1989.

Aristotle. *The Works of Aristotle Translated into English.* Ed. and trans. J. A. Smith and W. O. Ross. 12 vols. Oxford, 1908–1952.

Aron, M. L. "The Nature and Incidence of Stuttering among a Bantu Group of School-Going Children," *JSHD,* 27 (1962), 116–28.

Atherton, J. S. "Lewis Carroll and Finnegans Wake," *English Studies,* 33 (1952), 1–15.

Auden, W. H., and C. Isherwood. *The Ascent of F6.* London, 1938.

Bacon, Francis. *Sylva Sylvarum, or a Natural History in Ten Centuries.* 1627.

# Bibliography

Bandura, A. *Principles of Behavior Modification.* New York, 1969.

Barbara, D. A. *New Directions in Stuttering: Theory and Practice.* Springfield, IL, 1965.

———. *The Psychodynamics of Stuttering.* Springfield, IL, 1982.

Barber, V. "Studies in the Psychology of Stuttering: XV. Chorus Reading as a Distraction in Stuttering," *JSD,* 4 (1939), 371–83.

———. "Studies in the Psychology of Stuttering: XVI. Rhythm as a Distraction in Stuttering," *JSD,* 5 (1940), 29–42.

Barnett, G. L. *Charles Lamb.* Boston, 1976.

Barry, D. "Smoothing Out Stutters," *New York Daily News,* August 29, 1983, 13.

Barton, W. E. *The Life of Clara Barton, Founder of the American Red Cross.* 2 vols. New York, 1969.

Bede, the Venerable. *The Ecclesiastical History of the English People.* Trans. Leo Sherley-Price. London, 1955.

Beech, H., and F. Fransella. *Research and Experiment in Stuttering.* London, 1968.

Bell, A. *Stammering and Other Impediments of Speech.* London, 1836.

Belloc, H. *Charles the First, King of England.* Philadelphia, 1933.

Bender, J. F. *The Personality Structure of Stuttering.* New York, 1939.

Bennett, A. *The Letters of Arnold Bennett: A Portrait Done at Home.* London, 1935.

———. *Sketches for Autobiography.* Ed. James Hepburn. London, 1979.

Biddle, B. J., and E. J. Thomas (Eds.) *Role Theory: Concepts and Research.* New York, 1966.

Biggs, B. E., and J. G. Sheehan. "Punishment or Distraction? Operant Stuttering Revisited," *JAP,* 74 (1969), 256–62.

Birkenhead, Earl of. *Churchill, 1874–1922.* London, 1989.

Black, M. "Speech Correction in the USSR," *JSHD,* 25 (1960), 2–7.

Blainey, A. *Immortal Boy: A Portrait of Leigh Hunt.* London, 1985.

Blanton, Smiley, and Margaret Gray. *For Stutterers*. New York, 1936.

Bloodstein O. "The Anticipatory Struggle Hypothesis: Implications of Research on the Variability of Stuttering," *JSHR*, 15 (1972), 487–99.

———. *A Handbook on Stuttering*. National Easter Seal Society. Chicago, 1981.

———. "Stuttering as an Anticipatory Struggle Reaction," in J. Eisenson (Ed.), *Stuttering: A Symposium*. New York, 1958, 1–70.

———. "Stuttering as Tension and Fragmentation," in J. Eisenson (Ed.), *Stuttering: A Second Symposium*. New York, 1975.

———. *Stuttering: The Search for a Cause and Cure*. Boston, 1993.

Bloom, L. "Notes for a History of Speech Pathology," *Psychoanalytic Review*, 65 (1978), 433–63.

Bluemel, C. S. "Concepts of Stammering: A Century in Review," *JSHD*, 25 (1960), 24–32.

———. *Mental Aspects of Stammering*. Baltimore, 1930.

———. *The Riddle of Stuttering*. Danville, IL, 1957.

———. *Stammering and Cognate Defects of Speech*. New York, 1930.

Blunden, E. *Charles Lamb*. London, 1934.

Boas, R., and L. Boas. *Cotton Mather*. Hamden, CT, 1964.

Boberg, E. "The Winding Trails of Therapy: Convergence at Last," *The Speak Easy Newsletter*, 12, No. 2, 4–5.

Boberg, E. (Ed.) *Maintenance of Fluency: Proceedings of the Banff Conference*. New York, 1981.

——— (Ed.) *The Neuropsychology of Stuttering*. Edmonton, Alberta, 1993.

Boberg, E., and D. Kully. "A Retrospective Look at Stuttering Therapy," *Journal of Speech and Language Pathology*, 13 (1989). Reprinted by the Institute for Stuttering Treatment and Research, University of Alberta.

Boberg, E., and W. G. Webster. "Stuttering: Current Status of Theory and Therapy," *Canadian Family Physician*, 36 (1990), 1156–60.

# Bibliography

Boome, E. J., and M. A. Richardson. *The Nature and Treatment of Stuttering.* New York, 1932.

Bornfield, S. "Therapy Builds Confidence," *Gannett Westchester Newspapers,* January 29, 1987, C1–2.

Bowen, Elizabeth. *Pictures and Conversations.* Harmondsworth, Middlesex, 1975.

Bowle, J. *Charles I.* London, 1975.

Boyle, A. *The Fourth Man.* New York, 1979.

Brady, J. P. "The Pharmacology of Stuttering: A Critical Review," *AJP,* 148 (1991), 1309–16.

Brain, Walter Russell. *Speech Disorders.* London, 1961.

Bredif, L. *Demosthenes.* Chicago, 1881.

Breitweiser, M. R. *Cotton Mather and Benjamin Franklin.* London, 1984.

Brent, Peter. *Charles Darwin.* London, 1981.

Briggs, J., and R. Plutzig. "The Only Handicap That People Laugh At," *Parade Magazine,* August 24, 1986, 12.

Brodkey, Harold. Interview with author. February 15, 1993.

Brodribb, W. J. *Demosthenes.* London, 1877.

Brody, J. "Personal Health," *The New York Times,* June 23, 1982.

Brome, V. *Aneurin Bevan.* London, 1953.

Brookshire, R., and R. Eveslage. "Verbal Punishment of Disfluency Following Augmentation of Random Delivery of Aversive Stimuli," *JSHR,* 42 (1967), 383–88.

Brown, S. F. "Stuttering with Relation to Word Accent and Word Position," *JASP,* 33 (1938), 112–20.

Brutten, E. J. "Palmar Sweat Investigation of Disfluency and Expectancy Adaptation," *JSHR,* 6 (1963), 40–48.

Brutten, E. J., and D. Shoemaker. *The Modification of Stuttering.* Englewood Cliffs, NJ, 1967.

Bryngelson, B. "A Method of Stuttering," *JAP,* 30 (1935), 194–98.

———. "A Study of Laterality of Stutterers and Normal Speakers," *JSD,* 4 (1939), 231–36.

———. "The Stuttering Personality and Development," *NC,* 2 (1943), 162–71.

Bryngelson, B., and T. Clark. "Left-handedness and Stuttering," *Journal of Heredity,* 24 (1933), 387–90.

Burdin, G. "The Surgical Treatment of Stammering, 1840–1842," *JSHD,* 5 (1940), 43–64.

Burke, R. "Reduced Auditory Feedback and Stuttering," *Behavior Research and Therapy,* 7 (1969), 303–308.

Burr, H. G., and J. M. Mullendore. "Recent Investigations on Tranquilizers and Stuttering," *JSHD,* 25 (1960), 33–37.

Burt, F. D. *W. Somerset Maugham.* Boston, 1985.

Butcher, S. H. *Demosthenes.* London, 1911.

Calder, R. *Willie: The Life of W. Somerset Maugham.* London, 1989.

———. *W. Somerset Maugham and the Quest for Freedom.* New York, 1973.

Campbell, P. *My Life and Easy Times.* London, 1967.

Campbell, R. J. *Psychiatric Dictionary.* New York, 1981.

Carleton, C. *Charles I: The Personal Monarch.* London, 1983.

Carlisle, J. *Tangled Tongue: Living with a Stutter.* Toronto, 1985.

Carroll, L. *The Complete Works of Lewis Carroll.* London, 1939.

Cecil, D. *A Portrait of Charles Lamb.* London, 1983.

Chitty, S. *The Beast and the Monk: A Life of Charles Kingsley.* New York, 1975.

Churchill, R. S. *Winston S. Churchill: Young Statesman.* Boston, 1967.

———. *Winston S. Churchill: Youth.* London, 1966.

Cimorell-Strong, J. M., H. R. Gilbert, and J. V. Frick. "Dichotic Speech Perception: A Comparison Between Stuttering and Nonstuttering Children," *JFD,* 8 (1983), 77–91.

Clark, A. *Lewis Carroll.* London, 1979.

Collingwood, S. *The Life and Letters of Lewis Carroll (Rev. C. L. Dodgson).* London, 1898.

Collins, A. *Charles Kingsley.* London, 1950.

Columbat, M. *De bégaiement et de tous les autres vices de la parole.* Paris, 1830.

Compton, D. *Stammering*. London, 1993.

Conture, E. "Observing Laryngeal Movements of Stutterers," in W. H. Perkins, and R. F. Curlee (Eds.) *Nature and Treatment of Stuttering: New Directions*. San Diego, 1984.

Conture, E., G. McCall, and D. Brewer. "Laryngeal Behavior During Stuttering," *JSHR*, 20 (1977), 661–68.

Cooper, E. B. "Controversies About Stuttering Behavior," *JFD*, 2 (1977), 75–86.

———. Interviewed by Marilyn Newhoff. "Stuttering Nuggets from a Perennially Perplexed but Persevering Prospector," *The Clinical Connection*, 4 (1990), 2–4.

Cordell, R. A. *Somerset Maugham*. London, 1961.

Coriat, I. H. "The Psychoanalytic Conception of Stuttering," *NC*, 2 (1943), 167–71.

———. "Stammering—A Psychoanalytic Interpretation," *Nervous and Mental Diseases Monographs*, 47 (1928), 1–68.

Corner, George W. *Anatomical Texts of the Earlier Middle Ages*. Washington, DC, 1927.

Courtney, W. F. *Young Charles Lamb*. London, 1982.

Cox, N. J., R. A. Seider, and K. K. Kidd. "Some Environmental Factors and Hypotheses for Stuttering in Families with Several Stutterers," *JSHR*, 27 (1984), 543–48.

Craig, P. *Elizabeth Bowen*. New York, 1986.

Creighton, J. V. *Margaret Drabble*. London, 1985.

Croke, K. "Giving Voice to Their Fears," *New York Daily News*, August 18, 1988, 52.

Cross, D. E., and H. L. Luper. "Voice Reaction Time of Stuttering and Nonstuttering Children and Adults," *JFD*, 4 (1979), 59–77.

Cullinan, W. L., and M. T. Springer. "Voice Initiation Times in Stuttering and Nonstuttering Children," *JSHR*, 23 (1980), 344–60.

Cuniberti, B. "Annie Glenn Speaks Up," *Los Angeles Times*, 19, II, 2–3.

Curlee, R. and W. Perkins (Eds.) *Nature and Treatment of Stuttering: New Directions.* San Diego, CA, 1984.

Curry, F. K., and H. H. Gregory. "The Performance of Stutterers on Dichotic Listening Tasks Thought to Reflect Cerebral Dominance," *JSHR,* 12 (1969), 73–82.

Curtis, A. *The Pattern of Maugham.* New York, 1974.

Dalton, P. (Ed.) *Approaches to the Treatment of Stuttering.* London, 1983.

Daniels, E. M. "An Analysis of the Relation Between Handedness and Stuttering with Special Reference to the Orton-Travis Theory of Cerebral Dominance," *JSD,* 5 (1940), 309–26.

Darwin, C. *The Autobiography of Charles Darwin.* New York, 1964.

Darwin, E. *Zoonomia,* 2 vols. London, 1794–1796.

Darwin, F. (Ed.) *The Life and Letters of Charles Darwin.* Vol. 1. New York, 1896.

Day, R. *Larkin.* Philadelphia, 1987.

de Chegoin, H. *Recherches sur les causes et le traitement du bégaiement.* Paris, 1830.

De Keyser, J. "The Stuttering of Lewis Carroll," in *Neurolinguistic Approaches to Stuttering,* Y. Lebrun and R. Hoops, eds. Mouton, 1973.

Dickens, C. "Psellism: The Act of Stammering," *Household Words.* London (1856), 14.

Dieffenbach, J. F. *Die Heilung des Stotterns durch eine neue chirurgische Operation; ein Sendschreiben an das Institut von Frankreich.* Berlin, 1841.

D'Israeli, I. *Commentaries on the Life and Reign of Charles the First.* Vol. 1. London, 1828.

Drabble, M. *Arnold Bennett.* London, 1974.

Dugan A. *Poems.* New Haven, 1961.

Dunlap, K. "Stammering: Its Nature, Etiology and Therapy," *Journal of Comparative Psychology,* 37 (1944), 187–202.

Ecenbarger, W. "Speaking the Truth About Stuttering," *Express,* August 1987, 50–52.

———. "When Words Fail," *Philadelphia Inquirer,* May 31, 1987, 10–14, 23–24.

Eisenson, J. (Ed.) *Stuttering: A Symposium.* New York, 1958.

Eldridge, M. *A History of the Treatment of Speech Disorders.* Edinburgh, 1968.

*Encyclopaedia Britannica.* Chicago, 1988.

*Family Circle Magazine.* "The Ordeal of Annie Glenn." November, 1974.

Fisher, J. *My Darling Clementine.* London, 1960.

Foot, M. *Aneurin Bevan.* London, 1975.

Fortinberry, A. "Don't Abuse Your Voice," *Self,* March 1983.

Fraser, M. *Self-Therapy for the Stutterer.* Speech Foundation of America. Memphis, 1979.

Freeman, F. "Phonation in Stuttering: A Review of Current Research," *JFD,* 4 (1979), 78–89.

Freeman, F., and T. Ushijima. "Laryngeal Activity Accompanying the Moment of Stuttering: A Preliminary Report of EMG Investigations," *JFD,* 3 (1975), 36–45.

Freund, H. *Psychopathology and the Problems of Stuttering.* Springfield, IL, 1966.

Froeschels, E. "Survey of the Early Literature on Stuttering; Chiefly European," *NC,* 2 (1943), 86–95.

Galton, L. "Stuttering: A Full Cure?," *Parade Magazine,* September 21, 1980, 17.

Gardner, M. *The Annotated Alice: Alice's Adventures in Wonderland and Through the Looking Glass by Lewis Carroll.* London, 1964.

Garvin-Cullen, A. "The Relationship Between Locus-of-Control and the Effectiveness of Postremediation Activities on the Maintenance of Fluency." Doctoral dissertation. New York University, 1990.

Gattegno, J. *Lewis Carroll: Fragments of a Looking-Glass.* New York, 1974.

Glasner, P., and D. Rosenthal. "Parental Diagnosis of Stuttering in Young Children," *JSHD,* 22 (1957), 288–95.

Glauber, I. P. "The Psychoanalysis of Stuttering," in J. Eisenson, (Ed.), *Stuttering: A Symposium*. New York, 1958.

Glendinning, V. *Elizabeth Bowen*. New York, 1978.

Goodstein, L. D. "Functional Speech Disorders and Personality: A Survey of the Research," *JSHR*, 1 (1958), 359–76.

Graves, R. *I Claudius*. London, 1934.

Green, R. *The Story of Lewis Carroll*. London, 1949.

Greenacre, P. *Swift and Carroll*. New York, 1955.

Greene, J. S. and E. J. Wells. *The Cause and Cure of Speech Disorders*. New York, 1927.

Gregg, P. *King Charles I*. London, 1981.

Gregory, H. H. (Ed.) *Controversies About Stuttering Therapy*. Baltimore, 1979.

———— (Ed.) *Learning Theory and Stuttering Therapy*. Evanston, IL, 1968.

Gruber, L. "The Use of the Portable Voice Masker in Stuttering Therapy," *JSHD*, 1971 (36), 287–89.

Guitar, B. "Historic Treatments for Stuttering: From Pebbles to Psychoanalysis," *ASHA*, June–July 1989, 71.

————. "Is It Stuttering or Just Normal Language Development?," *Contemporary Pediatrics*, February 1988, 109–10, 113–16, 119, 122, 125.

————. "Pretreatment Factors Associated with the Outcome of Stuttering Therapy," *JSHR*, 19 (1976), 590–600.

————. "Reduction of Stuttering Frequency Using Analog Electromyographic Feedback," *JSHR*, 18 (1975), 672–85.

Guitar, B., and T. Peters. *Stuttering: An Integration of Therapies*. The Speech Foundation of America. Memphis, 1980.

Guttmann, O. *Gymnastics of the Voice for Song and Speech; Also a Method for the Cure of Stuttering and Stammering*. New York, 1893.

Gutzmann, A. *Das Stottern*. Berlin, 1890.

Hahn, E. F. *Stuttering: Significant Theories and Therapies*. Stanford, CA, 1950.

Hall, J., and J. Jerger. "Central Auditory Function in Stutterers," *JSHR,* 21 (1978), 324–37.

Hannley, M., and M. Dorman. "Some Observations on Auditory Function and Stuttering," *JFD,* 7 (1982), 93–108.

Haroldson, S. K., R. R. Martin, and C. D. Starr. "Time-out as a Punishment for Stuttering," *JSHR,* 11 (1968), 560–66.

Hassler, D. *Erasmus Darwin.* New York, 1973.

Helm, N. A., R. B. Butler, G. J. Cantor. "Neurogenic Acquired Stuttering," *JFD,* 5 (1980), 269–79.

Hepburn, J. G. *The Mind and Art of Arnold Bennett.* Ann Arbor, 1957.

Herodotus. *History.* Ed. and trans. A. D. Godley. London, 1924.

Hibbert, C. *Charles I.* New York, 1968.

Hippocrates. *The Medical Works of Hippocrates.* Ed. and trans. John Chadwick and W. N. Mann. Oxford, 1950.

Hoagland, E. *The Final Fate of the Alligators.* Santa Barbara, CA, 1992.

———. *Heart's Desire.* New York, 1988.

———. Interviews with author. August 17 and September 23, 1993.

Hogan, C. H. "Stuttering: What It Is, What It Isn't, and What Worked for Me," *MS,* May 1982, 36–38.

*Hollins Communications Research Institute.* "Fluency Master: A New Development for Those Who Stutter." Roanoke, VA, 1989.

Howie, P. M. "Concordance for Stuttering in Monozygotic and Dizygotic Twin Pairs, *JSHR,* 24 (1981), 317–21.

Hudson, D. *Lewis Carroll.* London, 1954.

———. *Lewis Carroll: An Illustrated Biography.* London, 1976.

Hunt, J. *Stammering and Stuttering, Their Nature and Treatment.* London, 1863. (Hafner facsimile, 1967.)

Hunt, Leigh. *The Autobiography of Leigh Hunt.* London, 1859.

Hutchinson, J. M., and B. M. Navarre. "The Effect of Metronome Pacing on Selected Aerodynamic Patterns of Stuttered Speech: Some Preliminary Observations and Interpretations," *JFD,* 2 (1977), 189–206.

Ickes, W. K., and S. Pierce. "The Stuttering Moment: A Plethysmographic Study," *JCD*, 6 (1973), 155–64.

*The Infinite Voyage.* "The Dawn of Humankind," transcript. QED Communications Inc. in association with the National Academy of Sciences. Kent, OH, 1992.

Ingham, R. J. "Evaluation and Maintenance in Stuttering Treatment: A Search for Ecstasy with Nothing but Agony," in E. Boberg (Ed.), *Maintenance of Fluency.* New York, 1981.

———. *Stuttering and Behavior Therapy: Current Status and Experimental Foundations.* San Diego, CA, 1983.

Ingham R. J., H. Southwood, and G. Horsburgh. "Some Effects of the Edinburgh Masker on Stuttering during Oral Reading and Spontaneous Speech," *JFD*, 6 (1981), 135–54.

Itard, J. M. "Traitement du bégaiement," *Journal Universel des Sciences Médicales,* 7 (1817), 129.

Jacobs, J. *History of the Aesopic Fable.* Burt Franklin reprint. New York, 1970.

Jaeger, W. W. *Demosthenes: The Origin and Growth of His Policy.* London, 1938.

James, R. R. *Churchill: A Study in Failure, 1900–1939.* London, 1970.

John, E. *King Charles I.* New York, 1950.

Johnson, R. B. *Leigh Hunt.* London, 1896.

Johnson, W. *Because I Stutter.* Iowa City, 1940.

———. "The Indians Have No Word for It. I. Stuttering in Children," *Quarterly Journal of Speech,* 30 (1944), 330–37.

———. *Stuttering and What You Can Do About It.* Minneapolis, 1961.

Johnson, W., and R. Leutenegger (Eds.). *Stuttering in Children and Adults.* Minneapolis, 1955.

Jonas, G. *Stuttering: The Disorder of Many Theories.* New York, 1976.

Jones, J. E. *Voices and Silences.* New York, 1993.

Joyce, J. *Finnegan's Wake.* New York, 1976.

Kanin, G. *Remembering Mr. Maugham.* London, 1966.

# Bibliography

Kaplan, F. *Henry James.* New York, 1992.

Kazin, A. *A Walker in The City.* New York, 1951.

Kenney, E. J., Jr. *Elizabeth Bowen.* London, 1975.

Kent L. R. "Carbon Dioxide Therapy as a Medical Treatment for Stuttering," *JSHD,* 26 (1961), 268–71.

———. "The Use of Tranquilizers in the Treatment of Stuttering," *JSHD,* 28 (1963), 288–94.

Kent L. R., and D. E. Williams. "Use of Meprobamate as an Adjunct to Stuttering Therapy," *JSHD,* 24 (1959), 64–69.

Kidd, K. K. "Genetic Models of Stuttering," *JFD,* 5 (1980), 187–201.

———. "A Genetic Perspective on Stuttering," *JFD,* 2 (1977), 259–69.

Kidd, K. K., R. C. Heimbeich, M. Records, G. Oehlert, and R. Webster. "Familial Stuttering Patterns Are Not Related to One Measure of Severity," *JSHR,* 21 (1978), 768–78.

Kidd, K. K., J. R. Kidd, and M. A. Records. "The Possible Causes of the Sex Ratio in Stuttering and Its Implications," *JFD,* 3 (1978), 13–23.

King-Hele, D. *Doctor of Revolution: The Life and Genius of Erasmus Darwin.* London, 1977.

Klingbeil, G. M. "Stuttering and Stammering," *JSD,* 4 (1939), 115–32.

Knightley, P. *Philby: The Life and Views of the K.G.B. Masterspy.* London, 1988.

Krause, E. *Erasmus Darwin. With a Preliminary Notice by Charles Darwin.* London, 1879.

Krug, M. M. *Aneurin Bevan: Cautious Rebel.* London, 1961.

Kupferberg, H. *The Mendelssohns: Three Generations of Genius.* New York, 1979.

LaFollette, A. C. "Parental Environment of Stuttering Children," *JSHD,* 21 (1956), 202–207.

Lamb, Charles. "Oxford in the Vacation," *Essays of Elia.* Eds. N. L. Hallward and S. C. Hill. London, 1960.

———. *The Works of Charles Lamb.* Ed. T. Hutchinson. Oxford, 1924.

Landers, A. "After Years of Unhappiness, Stutterers Overcome Handicap," *Providence Journal-Bulletin,* November 6, 1989.

Lassner, P. *Elizabeth Bowen.* London, 1990.

Lebrun, Y., and R. Hoops (Eds.) *Neurolinguistic Approaches to Stuttering.* Proceedings of the International Symposium on Stuttering (Brussels, 1972). The Hague, 1973.

Lee, B. S. "Artificial Stutter," *JSHD,* 16 (1951), 53–55.

Le May, M. "The Language Capability of Neanderthal Man," *American Journal of Physical Anthropology,* 42 (1975), 9–14.

Lemert, E. M. "Some Indians Who Stutter," *JSHD,* 18 (1953), 168–74.

———. "Stuttering and Social Structure in Two Pacific Societies," *JSHD,* 27 (1962), 3–10.

Lenaghan, R. T. (Ed.) *Caxton's Aesop.* Cambridge, MA, 1967.

*Letting Go.* Newsletter of the National Stuttering Project. San Francisco, 1980–1993.

Levin, D. *Cotton Mather.* Boston, 1978.

Lieberman, P., D. H. Klatt, and W. Wilson. "Vocal Tract Limitations on the Vowel Repertoires of Rhesus Monkey and Other Nonhuman Primates." *Science,* 164 (1969), 1185–87.

Loss, A. K. *W. Somerset Maugham.* New York, 1987.

Luper, H. (Ed.) *Stuttering: Successes and Failures in Therapy.* Speech Foundation of America. Memphis, 1968.

MacNamee, T. "Normativity in 18th Century Discourse on Speech," *JCD,* 17, No. 6 (1984), 407–23.

Maddison, R. E. W. *The Life of the Honourable Robert Boyle.* London, 1969.

Makuen, G. H. "Psychology of Stammering," *JNMD,* 43 (1941), 68–72.

Malebouche, F. *Précis sur les causes du bégaiement et sur les moyens de guérir.* Paris, 1841.

Mallard, A. R., and J. S. Kelley. "The Precision Fluency Shaping

Program: Replication and Evaluation," *JFD*, 7 (1982), 287–94.

Maraist, J. A., and C. Hutton. "Effects of Auditory Masking Upon the Speech of Stutterers," *JSHD*, 22 (1957), 385–89.

Markow-Totevy, G. *Henry James*. New York, 1969.

Martin, B. K. *Philip Larkin*. Boston, 1978.

Martin, R. R., and G. M. Siegel. "The Effects of Response Contingent Shock on Stuttering," *JSHR*, 9 (1966), 340–52.

———. "The Effects of Simultaneously Punishing Stuttering and Rewarding Fluency," *JSHR*, 9 (1966), 466–75.

Martin, S., and L. G. Hershey. "The Use of Haloperidol in the Management of Stuttering," *JFD*, 1 (1975), 13–17.

Mather, C. *The Angel of Bethesda*. Ed. G. W. Jones. Barre, MA, 1972.

———. *Diary*. 2 vols. Ed. W. Ford. Boston, 1911–12.

———. *Manuductio ad Ministerium*. Boston, 1726.

———. *Selections*. Ed. K. Murdock. New York, 1926.

Maugham, R. *Conversations with Willie*. London, 1978.

———. *Somerset and All the Maughams*. New York, 1966.

Maugham, S. "Arnold Bennett," in *Life and Letters*, June. London, 1931.

———. *Of Human Bondage*. London, 1915.

———. "Looking Back," *The Sunday Express* (London), September 9, 1962.

———. *Selected Works*. New York, 1955.

———. *The Summing Up*. London, 1938.

May, J. L. *Charles Lamb: A Study*. London, 1934.

Maycock, A. *Chronicles of Little Gidding*. London, 1954.

Melville, H. *Billy Budd and Other Tales*. New York, 1961.

Meyer, B. C. "Psychosomatic Aspects of Stuttering," *JNMD*, 101 (1945), 127–57.

Miller, B. *Leigh Hunt's Relations with Byron, Shelley and Keats*. New York, 1910.

Miller, D. "St-st-stuttering: It Isn't Hopeless," *Parade Magazine*, February 1982, 70–81.

Miller, P. (Ed.) *An Abyss Deep Enough.* New York, 1982.

Momigliano, Arnaldo. *Claudius the Emperor and His Achievement.* Oxford, 1934.

Moncour, J. P. "Parental Domination in Stuttering," *JSHD,* 17 (1952), 155–65.

Moore, W. E. "Hypnosis in a System of Therapy for Stutterers," *JSD,* 11 (1946), 117–22.

Moore, W. H., Jr., and E. Boberg. "Hemispheric Processing and Stuttering," in L. Rustin, H. Purser, and D. Rowley (Eds.) *Progress in the Treatment of Fluency Disorders.* London, 1987.

Morgan, T. *Churchill: Young Man in a Hurry.* New York, 1982.

———. *Maugham.* New York, 1980.

Morgenstern, J. J. "Socio-Economic Factors in Stuttering," *JSHD,* 21 (1956), 25–33.

Motion, A. *Philip Larkin: A Writer's Life.* New York, 1993.

Murray, F. P. *A Stutterer's Story.* Memphis, 1980.

Mysak, E. D. *Speech Pathology and Feedback Theory.* Springfield, IL, 1966.

Naik, M. K. *W. Somerset Maugham.* Norman, OK, 1966.

Neelley, J. "A Study of the Speech Behavior of Stutterers and Nonstutterers Under Normal and Delayed Auditory Feedback," *JSHD, Monograph Supplement,* 7 (1961), 63–82.

Nelson, S. E. "The Role of Heredity in Stuttering," *Journal of Pediatrics,* 14 (1939), 642–54.

Nelson, S. E., N. Hunter, and M. Walter. "Stuttering in Twins," *JSD,* 10 (1945), 335–43.

Neugebauer, W. "Program Offers Hope to Stutterers," *New York Daily News,* April 12, 1981, C1.

Newark, T. *Not Good at Talking.* London, 1985.

Nowack, W. J., and R. E. Stone. "Acquired Stuttering and Bilateral Cerebral Disease," *JFD,* 12 (1987), 141–46.

Nowell-Smith, S. (Ed.) *The Legend of the Master.* New York, 1948.

Nurnberg, H. G., and B. Greenwald. "Stuttering: An Unusual Side Effect of Phenothiazines," *AMJ,* (1981), 386–87.

# Bibliography

O'Neill, Ynez Viole. *Speech and Speech Disorders in Western Thought Before 1600.* Contributions in Medical History, Number 3. Westport, CT, 1980.

Otto, Catherine. Interview with author. December 16, 1993.

Page, B., D. Leitch, and P. Knightley. *Philby: The Man Who Betrayed a Generation.* London, 1977.

Page, N. (Ed.) *Henry James: Interviews and Recollections.* London, 1984.

Pakenham, P. *King Charles I.* London, 1950.

Parry, W. D. *Understanding and Controlling Stuttering: A Comprehensive New Approach Based on the Valsalva Hypothesis.* Privately printed. Merion, PA, 1992.

Patrusky, B. "The Secret Ben Can't Keep," *Stars and Stripes,* August 19, 1976, 14–17.

Peins, M. (Ed.) *New Approaches in Stuttering Therapy.* Boston, 1984.

Perkins, W. H. *Current Therapy in Communication Disorders: Stuttering Disorders.* New York, 1984.

———. "From Psychoanalysis to Discoordination," in H. Gregory (Ed.), *Controversies About Stuttering.* Baltimore, 1979.

———. "The Genesis of Heresy," *Hearsay,* the Journal of the Ohio Speech and Hearing Association, Fall 1986, 66–68.

Peters, T. J., and B. Guitar. *Stuttering: An Integrated Approach to Its Nature and Treatment.* Baltimore, 1991.

Philby, E. *Kim Philby: The Spy I Married.* New York, 1967.

Philby, K. *My Silent War.* London, 1969.

Pines, M. "Stuttering: Help Is on the Way," *The New York Times Magazine,* February 13, 1977.

Pirie, G. *Henry James.* Totowa, NJ, 1974.

Plutarch. *Lives.* Vol. 7. Trans. Bernadotte Perrin. London, 1928.

Polow, Nancy G. *A Stuttering Manual for the Speech Therapist.* Springfield, IL, 1975.

Pound, R. *Arnold Bennett.* London, 1952.

Prins, D., and R. J. Ingham. *Treatment of Stuttering in Early Childhood: Methods and Issues.* San Diego, 1983.

Prosek, R. A., A. A. Montgomery, B. E. Walden, and D. M. Schwartz. "Reaction-Time Measures of Stutterers and Nonstutterers," *JFD*, 4 (1979), 269–78.

Pryor, E. B. *Clara Barton: Professional Angel*. Philadelphia, 1987.

Quarrington, B. "Stuttering as a Function of the Information Value and Sentence Position of Words," *JAP*, 70 (1965), 221–24.

Raphael, F. *Maugham and His World*. London, 1976.

Rappoport, K. "Clinic Helps Actor Alleviate Stutter," *Indianapolis Star*, June 22, 1986.

Rieber, R. W. (Ed.) *The Problem of Stuttering: Theory and Therapy*. New York, 1977.

Rieber, R. W., and J. Wollock. "The Historical Roots of the Theory and Therapy of Stuttering," *JCD*, no. 10 (1977), 3–24.

Rochford, E. B. "Stutterers' Practices: Folk Remedies and Therapeutic Intervention," *JCD*, 16, no. 5 (1983), 373–84.

Rochford, E. B., and P. Johnstone. "Medieval Arabic Views on Speech Disorders: al-Razi (c. 865–925)," *JCD*, 12, no. 3 (1979), 229–43.

Ryan, B. P. "Stuttering Therapy in a Framework of Operant Conditioning and Programmed Learning," in H. H. Gregory (Ed.), *Controversies About Stuttering Therapy*. Baltimore, 1979.

Sadler, L. V. *Margaret Drabble*. Boston, 1986.

Savithri, S. R. "Speech and Hearing Science in Ancient India," *JCD*, 21, no. 4 (1988), 271–317.

———. "Speech Pathology in Ancient India—A Review of Sanskrit Literature," *JCD*, 20, no. 6 (1987), 437–45.

Schaubel, H. J., and R. F. Street. "Prostigmin and the Chronic Stutterer," *JSHD*, 14 (1949), 143–46.

Schwartz, M. *Stop Stuttering*. New York, 1986.

———. *Stuttering Solved*. Philadelphia, 1976.

Scramuzza, V. M. *The Emperor Claudius*. London, 1940.

Seale, P., and M. McConville. *Philby: The Long Road to Moscow*. London, 1973.

Seider, R. A., K. L. Gladstien, and K. K. Kidd. "Recovery and Persistence of Stuttering Among Relatives of Stutterers," *JSHD*, 48 (1983), 402–409.

Seward, A. *Memoirs of the Life of Dr. Darwin*. Philadelphia, 1804.

Shames, G., and D. Egolf. *Operant Conditioning and the Management of Stuttering*. Englewood Cliffs, NJ, 1976.

Shames, G., and C. Florence. *Stutter-Free Speech: A Goal for Therapy*. Columbus, OH, 1980.

Shames, G., and H. Rubin (Eds.). *Stuttering Then and Now*. Columbus, OH, 1986.

Shaw, C. K., and W. F. Shrum. "The Effects of Response-Contingent Reward on the Connected Speech of Children Who Stutter," *JSHD*, 37 (1972), 75–88.

Shearer, W. M., and F. B. Simmons. "Middle Ear Activity During Speech in Normal Speakers and Stutterers," *JSHR*, 8 (1965), 203–207.

Sheehan, J. G. "Conflict Theory of Stuttering," in J. Eisenson (Ed.), *Stuttering: A Symposium*, 121–66.

———. "Current Issues in Stuttering and Recovery," in H. H. Gregory (Ed.), *Controversies About Stuttering Therapy*. Baltimore, 1979.

———. "Stuttering as a Self-role Conflict," in H. H. Gregory (Ed.), *Learning Theory and Stuttering Therapy*. Evanston, IL, 1968.

——— (Ed.) *Stuttering: Research and Therapy*. New York, 1970.

Shute, N. *Slide Rule: The Autobiography of an Engineer*. New York, 1954.

Siegel, G. "Punishment, Stuttering, and Dysfluency," *JSHR*, 13 (1970), 677–714.

Siegel, G. M. "Moses the Stutterer," *Letting Go*, 7, 7–12.

Silverman, K. *The Life and Times of Cotton Mather*. New York, 1984.

Spadino, E. J. *Writing and Laterality Characteristics of Stuttering Children*. New York, 1941.

Starkweather, C. W. *Fluency and Stuttering*. Englewood Cliffs, NJ, 1987.

Starkweather, C.W., S. R. Gottwald, and M. M. Halfond. *Stuttering Prevention:A Clinical Method.* Englewood Cliffs, NJ, 1990.

Stevenson, L. G. "The Surgery of Stammering: A Forgotten Enthusiasm of the Nineteenth Century," *BHM,* 42 (1968), 527–54.

Stewart, J. L. "The Problem of Stuttering in Certain North American Indian Societies," *JSHD,* 1960, Monograph Supplement 6.

Suetonius. *The Twelve Caesars.* Trans. R. Graves. Middlesex, 1957.

Sutherland, R. *Language and Lewis Carroll.* The Hague, 1970.

Sutton, S., and R. Chase. "White Noise and Stuttering," *JSHR,* 4 (1961), 72.

Swan, M. *Henry James.* London, 1952.

Swinnerton, F. *Arnold Bennett:A Last Word.* London, 1978.

Thompson, C. O. *Robert Boyle: A Study in Biography.* Worcester, MA, 1882.

Thompson, J. R. *Leigh Hunt.* Boston, 1977.

Thorp, M. F. *Charles Kingsley, 1819–1875.* New York, 1969.

Thwaite, A. (Ed.) *Larkin at Sixty.* London, 1982.

Timms, D. *Philip Larkin.* Edinburgh, 1973.

Tolley, A. T. *My Proper Ground.* Carleton, Canada, 1991.

Townsend, P. *The Last Emperor.* London, 1975.

Travis, L. E. "The Cerebral Dominance Theory of Stuttering: 1931–1978," *JSHD,* 43 (1979), 278–81.

———. *Speech Pathology.* New York, 1931.

Updike, J. *Self-Consciousness: Memoirs.* New York, 1989.

Van Dantzig, M. "Syllable-tapping, a New Method for the Help of Stammerers," *JSD,* 5 (1940), 127–31.

Van Riper, C. "Experiments in Stuttering Therapy," in J. Eisenson (Ed.), *Stuttering:A Symposium.* New York, 1958.

———. "Historical Approaches to Stuttering," in J. G. Sheehan (Ed.), *Stuttering: Research and Therapy,* 36–54.

———. *The Nature of Stuttering.* Englewood Cliffs, NJ, 1971.

———. "Recollections from a Pioneer," *ASHA,* June-July 1989, 72.

————. *Speech Correction: Principles and Methods*. 4th ed. Englewood Cliffs, NJ, 1963.

Wada, J., and T. Rasmussen. "Intracarotid Injection of Sodium Amytal for the Lateralization of Cerebral Speech Dominance: Experimental and Clinical Observation," *Journal of Neurosurgery*, 17 (1960), 266–82.

Wall, M. J., and F. L. Myers. *Clinical Management of Childhood Stuttering*. Baltimore, 1984.

Wallace, R. *The Agony of Lewis Carroll*. Melrose, MA, 1990.

Walle, E. L. "Intracarotid Sodium Amytal Testing on Normal, Chronic Adult Stutterers," *JSHD*, 37 (1971), 561.

Watson, D. R. *The Life and Times of Charles I*. London, 1972.

Webster, R. L. "Empirical Considerations Regarding Controversies in Stuttering Therapy," in H. H. Gregory (Ed.), *Controversies About Stuttering Therapy*. Baltimore, 1978.

————. "Establishment of Fluent Speech in Stutterers." Paper presented at the American Association for the Advancement of Tension Control, in London, September 1979.

————. "Evolution of a Target-Based Behavioral Therapy for Stuttering," *JFD*, 5 (1980), 303–20.

————. Interviews with author. March 24, 1993, and May 11, 1994.

————. *The Precision Fluency Shaping Program: Speech Reconstruction for Stutterers*. 2 vols. Roanoke, VA, 1982.

Wepman, J. M. "Familial Incidence in Stammering," *JSD*, 4 (1939), 199–204.

West, R. "An Agnostic's Speculations About Stuttering," in J. Eisenson (Ed.), *Stuttering: A Symposium*. New York, 1958.

————. "Is Stuttering Abnormal?," *JAP*, 31 (1936), 76–86.

Westbrook, J. B. "Treatment—What's New? Fluency Aids," Special Interest Divisions, Fluency and Fluency Disorders, *ASHA*, 2 (August 1992), 1–7.

Wheeler-Bennett, J. W. *King George VI: His Life and Reign*. London, 1958.

Wijnen, F., and I. Boers. "Phonological Priming Effects in Stutterers," *JFD*, 19 (1994), 1–20.

Williams, D. E. "Stuttering Therapy: Where Are We Going and Why?," *JFD*, 7 (1982), 159–70.

Wingate, M. E. *Stuttering: Theory and Treatment*. New York, 1976.

Wollock, J. "Communication Disorders in Renaissance Italy: An Unreported Case Analysis by Hieronymus Mercurialis (1530–1606)," *JCD*, 23, no. 1 (1990), 1–30.

Wyllie, J. *The Disorders of Speech*. Edinburgh, 1894.

Zimmerman, G., S. Liljeblad, A. Frank, and C. Cleeland. "The Indians Have Many Terms for It: Stuttering Among the Bannock-Shoshoni," *JSHR*, 26 (1983), 315–18.

Zummo, S. "New Therapy for Stutterers," *Staten Island Advance*, April 24, 1981, B4.

# Index

Index

electronic measurement of stuttering, 169, 173
*Elements of Physics, and Natural Philosophy* (Arnott), 88
Elizabeth, Queen Mother, 147
Elizabeth I, Queen of England, 67
elocution, 77, 87, 91
environment, 132, 170
epiglottis, 26
epilepsy, 127
"Establishment of Fluent Speech in Stutterers, The" (Webster), 171
Euripides, 65
Evelyn, John, on Robert Boyle, 72
*Examiner,* 104
eyes:
    pupil enlargement in, 168
    squinting of, 94

face masks, 100
facial tics, 19
faith healing, 21
false-role disorder, 136
fear, 38, 121, 132, 169
*Fearful Majesty* (Bobrick), 176
Fear Survey Schedules, 168
feedback:
    auditory, 166–68, 172, 176, 177
    kinesthetic, 174–75
feeling, hearing of speech vs., 174
females:
    castration complex in, 124–25
    and competition theory, 133

and gender ratios, 18, 134, 170, 171
genetic risks of, 169
stuttering as becoming in, 18
fiber-optic films, 169
finger thumping, 45
*Finnegans Wake* (Joyce), 111
fixation theories, 21, 122–23
Flaubert, Gustave, 99
fluency:
    in chanting, 42
    in choral reading, 176
    devices for, 21, 85–86, 87, 177, 100
    in foreign languages, 42
    programs for, 173–74, 176
    and reading in unison, 42, 176
    and rhythm, 42, 77, 86, 87, 91–92, 101, 177
    in script reading, 40, 164
    in singing, 42, 59, 77, 91, 101, 176, 177
    in solitude, 101
    in whispering, 42, 101, 172, 176, 179
"Fluency Master," 177
foaming at the mouth, 19
Fontana (Tartaglia), Niccolò, 57–58
foot stamping, 19, 33–34
foreign languages, fluency in, 42
forks, for tongue support, 21, 85–86
four humors, doctrine of, 22, 53–54
Frank, Joseph, 87
frenum, division of, 52–53, 55, 86–87

Index

Freud, Sigmund, 122
  *see also* psychoanalysis
Froeschels, Emil, 122, 132

gadgets, therapeutic, 100
  forks, 21, 85–86
  isochromes, 86
  muthonomes, 87
Galen, 51–52
gargles, 54
gasping, 19
gender ratios, 18, 134, 169, 170,
  171
Genesis, 23
genetics, 101, 169–70, 171
gentle onset, 83
  targets for, 173–74
George III, King of England, 79
George VI, King of England,
  146–48, 154, 155
Glenn, Annie, 164–65
glottis, *see* tongue
goat feces, 87
Goldsmith, Oliver, 43
Gosse, Edmund, on Henry
  James, 113
grammar, as innate, 25
Graves, Robert, on Claudius I,
  69
Greece, ancient:
  language philosophy in,
    23–24
  speech pathology in, 22,
    49–51
Greene, J. S., 32
Guttman, Oskar, 132

habitual stuttering, 60–61, 87,
  90, 102, 128
Hahn, Johann Gottfried, 61

Hall, Marshall, 87–88
haloperidol, 171
handedness, left or right, 126,
  179
hard palate, 27
Harlow, Clarissa (Clara Barton),
  118–19, 155
Harrison, John, 182
Hayes, Lester, 44, 169
head injury, 30
hearing:
  and auditory feedback,
    166–68, 172, 176, 177–78
  vs. feeling, 174
heart rate, 168
Heinlein, Robert, 44
hemispheric dominance, cerebral, 126–27, 129, 131,
  179–80
herbal remedy, 57
heredity, 84, 101, 169–70, 171
Herodotus, 50
Herrick, Robert, 62
Hildanus, Fabricius, 53
Hippocrates, 51, 185
Hoagland, Edward, 31, 38, 139,
  153–54, 184
Hollins Communications Research Institute (Roanoke,
  Va.), 164, 175
Hollins Precision Fluency
  Shaping Program, 173–74,
  175, 181
Holme, Randle, 93–94
home environment, 132
Homer, 49
homosexuality, 124
Horace, 18
*Household Words,* 23
humidity, in brain, 54

Printed in the United States
By Bookmasters